The End of Roe v. Wade

Inside the Right's Plan to Destroy Legal Abortion

Robin Marty
Jessica Mason Pieklo

PUBLISHING

New York, NY

Printed in the United States of America.
10 9 8 7 6 5 4 3 2 1

The End of Roe V. Wade is an updated edition of *Crow After Roe*, previously published by Ig Publishing in 2013.

Ig Publishing
Box 2547
New York, NY 10163

www.igpub.com

ISBN: 978-1-632460-85-1 (paperback)

CONTENTS

Introduction

THE DAY THE END BEGAN

On June 27, 2018, there was no indication on that the abortion rights landscape was about to undergo a seismic shift to the right. That morning, the Supreme Court was finishing up another contentious term, releasing a decision undercutting the power of public sector unions to collect dues and using the First Amendment to justify its decision. Just the day before, the conservatives on the Court had upheld President Donald Trump's Muslim travel ban, and earlier in the month, had punted on resolving a case involving a Colorado baker who had refused to bake a cake for a same-sex couple because of a religious objection to marriage equality.

But with no abortion rights cases on the Court's docket for the following term, and still feeling optimistic about the previous year's abortion rights win in *Whole Woman's Health v. Hellerstedt,* pro-choice advocates turned their attention to challenging a fresh new wave of anti-abortion measures in the states. The ascendency of Donald Trump and Mike Pence to the presidency in 2016 had emboldened the religious right, who saw this as their moment to realize over forty years of grassroots and institutional advocacy to overturn *Roe v. Wade*. Yet as the Court's term came to a close that early summer day, anti-abortion forces didn't realize just how close they were to achieving their dream.

After the Court finished its business, the reports started coming in. Supreme Court Justice Anthony Kennedy, the Court's swing vote and the Justice widely believed to be the key vote to keeping *Roe* on the books, was retiring. President Trump, who had campaigned on a promise of only appointing Supreme Court justices intent on overturning *Roe*, would get to name Kennedy's replacement.

And just like that, the pendulum on abortion rights had swung back sharply in the anti-abortion movement's favor.

•

"Liberty finds no refuge in a jurisprudence of doubt," wrote Justice Sandra Day O'Connor in the opening of *Planned Parenthood v. Casey*, the 1992 abortion rights decision that would both re-affirm *Roe's* holding that the right to an abortion is fundamental, and also adopt the "undue burden" standard for judging future abortion restrictions. "The woman's liberty is not so unlimited, however, that from the outset the State cannot show concern for the life of the unborn, and at a later point in the fetal development the State's interest in life has sufficient force so that the right of the woman to terminate the pregnancy can be restricted," O'Connor's opinion in *Casey* continued. The undue burden formula in *Casey* shifted the Court's intellectual framework away from considering abortion to be a fundamental right upon which the State should carefully intrude, to abortion as a right that existed only in relation to the power of the state to regulate it.

Justice Anthony Kennedy was only in his fourth year on the Court when *Casey* was decided. A centrist from California, Kennedy had been appointed by President Ronald Reagan to replace the retired Justice Lewis F. Powell, Jr. Kennedy wasn't Reagan's first choice; former Nixon Solicitor General and culture warrior Robert Bork was the president's initial pick. Reagan, a conservative Republican, was a staunch opponent of abortion rights and his rise to the presidency opened a new era of political power for social conservatives. But it was Bork's fierce, public opposition to abortion rights and civil rights that would doom his nomination and ultimately put Kennedy on the bench. Had Bork been confirmed, it is very likely that *Casey* would have been decided the other way, with *Roe* possibly being overturned within twenty years of having been decided in 1973. But instead it was Justice Kennedy joining O'Connor to save *Roe v. Wade*, and abortion rights supporters breathed a sigh of relief—at least for a little while.

If O'Connor had hoped her opinion in *Casey* would end the question of whether or not *Roe* was settled law, that hope could not have lasted long. *Casey's* undue burden framework gave anti-abortion advocates a new opening in their war on choice. Individual states were now free to test the limits of what constituted an undue burden on abortion rights.

And test the limits they have. In the last decade, states controlled by Republican lawmakers have become laboratories to cook up the most restrictive, yet constitutionally acceptable, limitations on abortion rights under *Casey*. States that were once without mandatory waiting periods saw bills mandating a twenty-four-hour waiting period between a consultation with a doctor and the actual termination of a pregnancy. Those that already had one-day waiting periods saw that period extended to three days. States that allowed minors to obtain abortions without involving their parents were now ordering girls to notify their parents in advance, while those that already had parental notification laws in place were now proposing parental consent, sometimes from both parents, as well as limiting the ability to obtain a judicial bypass. Dozens of states have made getting an ultrasound as well as listening to a government-sponsored script describing the image and warning about the possibility of depression, suicide, breast cancer and other medically disproven "side effects" of abortion a prerequisite to termination. Others forbid abortion prior to viability of the fetus even if the fetus has a terminal condition or the patient's health is at risk. States are placing more and more limitations on medications used to cause an abortion. In at least five states, access has whittled down to a single clinic.

This and more have been the end result of a right-wing campaign that began the day *Roe v. Wade* was decided in January 1973. And with the election of Donald Trump, the retirement of Justice Anthony Kennedy and Brett Kavanaugh's ascension to replace him, this campaign is now about to bring us to the end of *Roe v. Wade*.

1

WHERE IT ALL STARTED

NEBRASKA, "THE GOOD 'LIFE'"

Since the 1970's a sign proclaiming "The Good Life" welcomes you into Nebraska, a land of cornfields, the College World Series, and an unwavering belief by many of its residents that just as there is no contradiction in being a registered Democrat who hasn't voted against a Republican candidate in decades, there is also no contradiction in believing the government's interference should be outlawed in every instance except when it comes to a person's right to choose to end a pregnancy.

So when State Senator Danielle Conrad stood in the front of the state's unicameral legislature in Lincoln, Nebraska in March 2010, she no doubt knew she was already the champion of a lost cause. The "Pain-Capable Unborn Child Protection Act," a new and unprecedented piece of legislation introduced by Nebraska Senator (and Speaker of the Legislature) Mike Flood and extensively advocated for by Nebraska Right to Life, the state's powerful anti-abortion lobbying group, had already been sponsored by 22 members of the legislature—nearly half of its 49 senators. Even if she couldn't defeat the bill, Conrad wanted to at least expose the medical fallacies, distortions and legal issues residing in its language, as well as its intent to try to end abortion under the guise of "saving babies from excruciating pain." "It was important to create a legal record," Conrad said, explaining why she put so much effort into countering the bill. "If Nebraska Right to Life supports a bill it is going to become law. But it needed to be shown that there was not unanimous consent, that the evidence presented wasn't undisputed, and the variety of issues that weren't being taken into account when the law was crafted."[1]

In many ways, Nebraska was an obvious choice to fire the opening shot in the battle to overturn *Roe v. Wade*, as the state offered several major advantages when it came to testing a piece of model anti-abortion legislation before it got fed to other restriction-friendly states across the country. First, due to Nebraska's unicameral legislature, the "Pain-Capable Unborn Child Protection Act" would only require one body to vote it through, eliminating the potential for it to be derailed by critics or watered down with amendments in a compromise between the House and Senate. Also, the smaller number of lawmakers to woo, many of whom already opposed abortion in nearly every circumstance, made passage of the bill certain, something the Right to Life activists needed in order to build their momentum as they began their push to challenge *Roe*. The hearings on the bill would provide them a platform to debate their talking points on a fetus's alleged ability to feel pain, their justification for why *Roe v. Wade* should be reviewed and reconsidered.

Furthermore, there was the added bonus of potentially eliminating the practice of Dr. LeRoy Carhart. A long-term provider of abortions in Nebraska, Carhart became the sole practitioner to openly perform later term abortions in the Midwest after the 2009 murder of Dr. George Tiller in Kansas. A thorn in the side of anti-abortion activists in the Cornhusker state since the late 1980s, Carhart had fought vehemently against restrictions meant to undermine a pregnant person's ability to access an abortion, including parental notification laws and bans on certain types of later term abortion procedures. Anti-abortion forces had been trying for years to get Carhart to close up shop. On the day that a parental notification law was passed in 1991, for example, Carhart was the victim of a mysterious fire at his farm, killing many of his horses and a few house pets.[2] While the fire department said it could not determine the cause of the blaze, a letter Carhart received the following day at his clinic took credit for the fire and blamed it on his performing abortions. It was that act of violence that turned Carhart from a doctor who provided abortions into an unapologetic activist.

In 2000, Carhart filed his first lawsuit to try and halt Nebraska's attempts to restrict abortion, suing the state for outlawing a type of procedure used primarily in later term abortions. Dubbed "partial birth abortion" by abortion foes, the term referred to an "intact D&E", but was vague enough to potentially criminalize any type of dilation and extraction (D&E) abortion, a type of abortion performed usually once the patient is fourteen weeks or beyond. In an additional affront to the right to choose, the bill also took a direct and determined swing at *Roe v. Wade* by not allowing an exception for the health of the pregnant person. The reason, according to the state legislature, was that there is no such thing as a medically necessary abortion.

Carhart brought suit against Don Stenberg, who was then the Republican Attorney General of Nebraska, challenging the partial birth ban on several fronts, including the lack of a health exception. Carhart argued that without such an exception, the law failed even the lowered "undue burden" standard for permissible abortion restrictions first articulated in a dissenting opinion by Justice Sandra Day O'Connor in *Akron v. Akron Center for Reproductive Health* and later adopted in *Planned*

Parenthood v. Casey. Those cases ruled that states were allowed to put "reasonable" restrictions on pre-viability abortions as long as they did not place extreme hardship on patients trying to obtain them.

Carhart's challenge was successful in federal district court as well as in an appeal filed in the Eighth Circuit Court of Appeals. When the Supreme Court agreed to review the lower court decisions, it represented one of the first true tests of the *Casey* "undue burden" standard as well as an opportunity to survey the cultural shift in the high court away from viewing abortion access as a component of a pregnant person's liberty and toward protecting the liberty of potential fetal life.

Justice Stephen Breyer delivered the majority decision in *Stenberg v. Carhart*, striking down the Nebraska law, but it ultimately turned out not to be the victory pro-choice advocates had hoped for, as the decision established a legal standard that would later be leveraged by conservatives to chip away at the ability to access abortion care. Citing *Casey*, Breyer wrote that any abortion law that imposed an "undue burden" on the "right to choose" was unconstitutional and that, in this case, the Nebraska law failed because it caused those who sought or procured abortion to fear prosecution, conviction and imprisonment. Though it was not apparent at the time, the focus of the Court's analysis had permanently shifted, as no longer would it first consider the individual liberty rights of a patient. Instead, it would assume a legitimate state interest in protecting fetal rights, then balance the pregnant person's rights against that. Those who were carrying the pregnancy had officially become the secondary consideration in the restrictions on abortion access.

Justices Ruth Bader Ginsberg and Sandra Day O'Connor each wrote concurring opinions. Ginsberg's concurrence stated unequivocally that the state could not force physicians to use procedures other than those they felt were safe based on their own judgment and training. Importantly, she tied this prohibition on state action to the individual "life and liberty" protection under the Constitution. It was an analytical framework Breyer had either accidentally or intentionally disregarded in his majority opinion. Justice O'Connor agreed with Ginsberg's concurrence and reinforced that any law that sought to regulate out of existence a particular medical procedure would have to be applied only to prevent unnecessary partial-birth abortions, and would have to include an exception for the health of the pregnant person. Since the Nebraska law did not, O'Connor said it could not stand.

Justice Antony Kennedy wrote the Court's dissenting opinion, arguing that the Nebraska ban was permitted under *Casey* and that the state had a legitimate interest in protecting prenatal life. Because the State of Nebraska had concluded that "partial-birth" abortions were never medically necessary, Kennedy argued there could be no "undue burden" on a person's "right to choose" since no one would never be in a position to "choose" this procedure in an emergency. The rest of the conservative wing of the court added predictably blistering dissents. Justice Antonin Scalia even referred back to his earlier dissent in the *Casey* ruling, calling the standard "unprincipled" in its origin and "doubtful" in its application. Scalia wrote that he believed not only this case, but also *Casey*—and by implication *Roe*—should be overturned, suggesting that "undue burden" was so broad as to allow pro-choice activists to claim any regulation of abortion would be "burdensome," making states unable to hyper-regulate abortion. It was an argument that turned both logic and decades of constitutional jurisprudence on its head.

While the Court ultimately struck down the Nebraska partial birth ban by a 5 to 4 majority, the victory for pro-choice advocates would be short-lived. Over the next ten years, a more conservative Supreme Court, an entirely different Department of Justice and a repudiation of decades of legal precedent would reveal just how tenuous the basic protections of *Roe* had become.

•

In November 2003, Republican President George W. Bush signed into law the federal Partial-Birth Abortion Ban Act, a copycat version of the law that had been struck down as unconstitutional in Nebraska three years earlier. It was challenged almost immediately by abortion-rights advocates, including Planned Parenthood and LeRoy Carhart. Because of the near-identical nature of the two pieces of legislation, several lower courts, including the Eighth Circuit, found the Partial-Birth Abortion Ban Act unconstitutional, relying on the reasoning and the precedent established in *Stenberg*. When the Supreme Court agreed to review the case in 2006, it became clear it wanted to revisit *Stenberg*, if only to address the differences between states enacting specific abortion procedure bans and the federal government doing so. By this time, the Court had become more conservative then the one that had ruled on *Stenberg* just a few years prior, primarily because Justice Sandra Day O'Connor had retired and been replaced by abortion foe Samuel Alito. With this change in its makeup, the new court made it clear it wanted an opportunity to revisit abortion rights, and the Bush administration's top lawyer, Alberto Gonzales, was going to make sure it had its chance.

Justice Kennedy wrote the majority opinion in *Gonzales v. Cahart*, upholding the constitutionality of the partial-birth ban and ruling that Dr. Carhart and Planned Parenthood had failed to show that Congress lacked authority to outlaw this specific abortion procedure. Abortion had once again become an area of federal concern; despite the Supreme Court's increasing interest in limiting the power of the federal government, when it came to abortion, the conservative justices had no issue with Congress prohibiting specific medical procedures and dictating practices to doctors across the country. Furthermore, once again showing a willingness to defer to legislative assertions that intact D&E abortions were never needed to protect the health of a pregnant person, Kennedy also held that a health exception was unnecessary—correcting what the anti-abortion wing of the Court perceived as the greatest flaw in the *Stenberg* decision. The Court also determined that Congress was entitled to regulate in an area where the medical community has not reached a "consensus," thus granting anti-abortion foes an opening to drive the "evidence" behind legislation targeting reproductive health care and choice.

Most distressing of all, the Court decided to "assume . . . for the purposes of this opinion" that the principles of *Roe v. Wade* and *Planned Parenthood v. Casey* governed. In other words, the majority signaled that *Roe* and *Casey* were in effect . . . for the moment. For court watchers everywhere, this was a visible and blatant signal to anti-abortion forces that *Roe* could be overturned in its entirety by the Court if the right case were brought before it. Justice Kennedy wrote that he believed the lower courts had wrongly decided a central premise of *Casey* in ruling that a pregnant person's right to choose abortion superseded a state's ability to place burdens on abortion in the interest of preserving fetal life. Since the federal ban fit that state interest, Kennedy wrote, it did not create an undue burden on the right to choose. Kennedy held that "ethical and moral concerns," including an interest in fetal life, represented "substantial" state interests which could be a basis for legislation at all times during pregnancy, not just after viability as posited in *Roe* and limited in *Casey*. This effectively erased the pre-viability/post-viability distinction and rendered meaningless any previous understanding of how an "undue burden" on a right to chose would be measured.

However, it was in its explanation of its abandonment of *Stenberg* where the conservative shift in the Court became most apparent. The Court held that the state statute at issue in *Stenberg* was more ambiguous than the later federal statute at issue in *Carhart*, despite the nearly identical language and findings supporting both laws. More strikingly, the majority avoided all previous abortion case precedent by not analyzing the federal ban under a "due process" standard. Instead, they simply stated that the Court disagreed with the conclusion of the Eighth Circuit that the federal statue conflicted with due process considerations, without explaining how it arrived at this conclusion.

Justice Ruth Bader Ginsberg led the dissent, joined by justices David Souter, John Paul Stevens and Stephen Breyer. She argued passionately that the ruling was an "alarming" one that ignored Supreme Court abortion precedent and "refuse[d] to take *Casey* and *Stenberg* seriously." Referring in particular to the Court's holding in *Casey*, Ginsberg sought to re-ground the Court's abortion jurisprudence in its previous acceptance of women's autonomy and equal citizenship rather than the more nebulous and shifting previous approach centering around privacy. "Thus," she wrote, "legal challenges to undue restrictions on abortion procedures do not seek to vindicate some generalized notion of privacy; rather, they center on a woman's autonomy to determine her life's course, and thus to enjoy equal citizenship stature." Due process cannot be ignored, according to Ginsberg, unless the Court disregards women as full and equal citizens under the law.

Ginsberg also took issue with the lack of a health exception in the federal ban, writing that "the absence of a health exception burdens all women for whom it is relevant—women who, in the judgment of their doctors, require an intact D&E because other procedures would place their health at risk." In general, her dissent criticized the usurpation of medical decision-making by legislators and the minimization of "the reasoned medical judgments of highly trained doctors . . . as 'preferences' motivated by 'mere convenience.'" While Justice Kennedy's majority opinion in *Carhart* did not explicitly overrule *Roe* or *Casey*, in her dissent, Ginsberg made it clear that it might as well have. "*Casey's* principles, confirming the continuing vitality of 'the essential holding of *Roe*,' are merely 'assume[d]' for the moment . . . rather than 'retained' or 'reaffirmed.'" Ginsberg concluded by criticizing the majority for abandoning the principle of stare decisis, writing that "a decision so at odds with our jurisprudence should not have staying power."

But staying power is exactly what the *Carhart* decision had.

•

By 2010, emboldened by an explicitly sympathetic Supreme Court, with John Roberts having replaced William Rehnquist as Chief Justice (while he joined with the anti-abortion wing of the Court, Rehnquist had not been a judicial conservative the caliber of Roberts), anti-abortion activists turned their attention to their next crusade: fetal pain. The "Pain-Capable Unborn Child Protection Act," like many abortion restrictions, was created by anti-abortion activists and lawyers as a piece of model legislation that could be fed to friendly legislators to propose in local governments across the country—in particular, conservative, abortion-restriction loving states in the Midwest and South.

Written by lawyers from the National Right to Life Committee, the Pain-Capable Unborn Protection Act was considered the next logical step in "fetal pain" legislation, building off a 2003 Minnesota law that mandated that abortion providers must offer those seeking abortions the following statement, "Some experts have concluded the unborn child feels physical pain after 20 weeks gestation. Other experts have concluded pain is felt later in gestational development. This issue may need further study." Further study was in fact done, with a 2005 article in the *Journal of the American Medical Association* concluding that, after reviewing multiple studies, "Evidence regarding the capacity for fetal pain is limited but indicates that fetal perception of pain is unlikely before the third trimester."[3, 4] Despite this finding, Nebraska Speaker Mike Flood, one of the state's most actively anti-abortion senators, introduced the Pain-Capable Unborn Child Protection Act at the end of January of 2010, prioritizing a bill Nebraska Right to Life called their "priority legislation for 2010."[5]

A young senator who had quickly made a name for himself as a politician to watch, Flood was named to *Time* magazine's "40 under 40" list in 2010 as part of "a new generation of civic leaders . . . already at work trying to fix a broken system and restore faith in the process."[6] Elected in 2004 from Norfolk, Nebraska, and becoming Speaker just three years later, Flood claimed that he wrote the Pain-Capable bill not to try to stoke a challenge to *Roe*, but "to stop Dr. LeRoy Carhart of Bellevue from becoming the region's main provider of late-term abortions."[7] Mary Spaulding Balch, the State Legislative Director for National Right to Life in Nebraska, was more blunt about the intentions of the bill. "I think National Right to Life wants to see something go to the Supreme Court that would provide more protection to the unborn child," she told the *Omaha Word Herald* in February, 2010. "What I would like to bring to the attention of the court is, there is another line. This new knowledge is something the court has not looked at before and should look at."[8]

Introduced on January 21, 2010, the Pain-Capable Unborn Protection Act was declared a priority bill on February 19, allowing it to fast track through the unicameral legislature. Senator Conrad, who became the face of opposition for the bill, filed numerous amendments to try to add exceptions for fetal anomaly and health of the pregnant person, all of which were defeated. Only one change to the ban ultimately made it through—an allowance for abortion in the case that the procedure could save the life of a surviving child in utero. This extremely narrow exception was created to address the testimony of Tiffany Campbell, a South Dakota woman who discovered late in her pregnancy that her fetuses suffered from a rare condition known as twin to twin transfusion syndrome. Fetuses with this syndrome are identical twins who, due to chromosomal issues, share a placenta with abnormal blood vessels that connect the umbilical cord and the shared circulatory system of the twins. It is a condition that in its most severe cases can kill both fetuses before birth. According to Campbell, one twin's heart was doing the work for both twins, and the effort of driving blood through both bodies was weakening him to the point where both would die. As her husband Chris explained to *NPR* in 2009, "Brady's heart was doing all the work. He was pumping all the blood, and he was starting to show the effects of the strain . . . and he was really at severe risk of cardiac arrest."[9]

After meeting with several doctors, it was determined that the only option was to abort the second twin, allowing the first twin's heart to do less work and keep Tiffany out of danger, too. "It was awful," Tiffany told reporters. "How do you give up on one of your children? But we were forced to make a decision. We don't regret our decision. We regret having to make that decision to choose one child over the other. We live . . . every single day with what we did. But then we look at Brady and say, 'Wow, he would not be here otherwise.'"[10]

After that experience, Campbell began testifying at anti-abortion hearings, explaining the real-life consequences of restrictions that don't take into account the medical condition of the fetus unless the person carrying it is truly in imminent danger of losing her life. She spoke out first against South Dakota's proposed full abortion ban ballot initiative in

2008, and two years later at the Nebraska fetal pain hearing. "We could let nature run its course and pray miraculously by the grace of God that both our boys would survive or we could abort the sicker of the two and give one of our sons a fighting chance to survive. We decided to abort one of our sons at 22 weeks" she told the legislature during one of many days of testimony on the bill.[11]

While the exception allowed patients in Campbell's situation to choose an abortion, it did not offer any such protections for pregnant people whose fetuses had other life-threatening complications. Those whose fetuses had severe birth defects, for example, would not have the same option, despite the low likelihood of survival after birth. There was no exception for fetuses with anencephaly, a neural tube disorder that causes a fetus to grow despite missing part or all of its brain, a condition that is incompatible with life even if the baby survives birth. There was also no exception for fetuses with trisomies, many of which create fatal defects of the heart that would force those fetuses who did survive outside the womb to live short, painful lives for the hours or days they would be on life support. There was no exception for fetuses with severe gastroschisis, a condition where a fetus's intestines grow outside the abdominal cavity and need to be surgically inserted back inside the abdomen via surgery after birth, even though the organs are sometimes so damaged that they cannot be repaired. Most importantly, the law did not allow a medical exception for cases like that of Dawn Mosher, whose fetus was diagnosed with the most severe form of spina bifida possible, another neural tube disorder in which the spinal canal doesn't fuse closed.[12] Should her fetus have survived its birth, (Dawn had an abortion), its short life would have been filled with the kind of suffering that Flood, his supporters and the National Right to Life movement claimed they created the bill to protect babies from feeling.

Although exceptions for non-viable fetuses were proposed during the hearings on the bill, Flood shot them all down, saying that although he did not want to "hurt people" with his ban, all fetuses are humans who deserve to be born, whatever "disabilities" they had. "I also ask the question, why does a baby that's going to be born with a disability become a better candidate for an abortion? Does their disability make them less human? Are they less deserving of the state's protection?" [13] Conrad quickly rebuked the Speaker. "We are not talking about engineering perfect pregnancies. We are talking about pregnancies incompatible with life." [14]

The testimony for the first fetal pain bill in the country set the stage for what would become the basic pattern in every other state that proposed legislation based on the same model. Abortion opponents would first present "evidence" that a fetus could feel pain by twenty weeks, providing testimony from expert witnesses to support that claim. In Nebraska, that evidence came from Dr. Jean Wright, Chair of Pediatrics at Mercer University School of Medicine, and Dr. Kanwaljeet (Sunny) Anand of Arkansas Children's Hospital Research Institute and the University of Arkansas College of Medicine. Dr. Wright had been a featured speaker at the Focus on the Family Conference of Medical Professionals and Spouses in 2008.[15] A "traditional family values" organization launched in 1977 by Dr. James Dobson, Focus on the Family is against women working outside the home, abortion in any form and even some types of contraception they claim are "abortifacient"—an erroneous belief that said contraception can cause a fertilized egg to not implant in the womb. By 2010, Wright and Anand had become the go to sources when it came to using fetal pain as a basis of passing anti-abortion laws. Both had testified in front of Congress to support the Partial Birth Abortion Ban Act, using their experiences in dealing with micro-preemies and surgery done in utero as a basis for claims that a fetus could feel "extreme" pain by at the latest twenty weeks post-gestation.

As evidence of their assertion, Wright and Anand referred to fetuses in utero "recoiling" from needles, or an increase in stress hormones that quantified fear and pain. However, most mainstream medical professionals consider these reactions to be involuntary reflexes that cannot be attributed to actual experience of pain since they can be seen in patients in vegetative states as well.[16] National Right To Life's Spaulding summarized this "expert" medical testimony to *LifeNews*. "By 20 weeks after fertilization, unborn children have pain receptors throughout their body, and nerves link these to the brain. These unborn children recoil from painful stimulation, which also dramatically increases their release of stress hormones. Doctors performing fetal surgery at and after 20 weeks now routinely use fetal anesthesia."[17]

Ironically, within a matter of years the very same doctor whose testimony was used to push the first "fetal pain" bans into passage would later come to qualify his own lack of support for the bans themselves. In 2013, when the bills began making national headlines, Anand told *The New York Times* that while he still believed a fetus likely felt pain at eighteen to twenty-four weeks, he believed "fetal pain does not have much relevance for abortion, since most abortions are performed before the fetus is capable of experiencing pain," and that for the "very few" abortions that were occurring after that point in gestation it would be simple to use other means to prevent pain rather than banning the abortions outright. He also said that he had been asked many times to testify in hearings to ban abortion and had refused.[18]

In Nebraska, however Wright and Anand's evidence that pre-term babies in neonatal intensive care units often react to IVs and shots by crying or turning away was then followed by a litany of rhetoric from supporters of the bill in the legislature. A few senators apologized that they could not eliminate abortion altogether but praised the bill as an excellent "first step." One senator declared that people on both sides needed to stop using the "F word" (i.e. fetus) because it was "offensive and demeaning." "He/she is an unborn child," he said. "He is someone's son. She is someone's daughter. He is someone's grandson. She is someone's granddaughter."[19]

The hearings grew even testier as senators began to debate the lack of a mental health exception to the bill. The omission was especially noticeable because Nebraska was concurrently debating and passing a bill that would mandate abortion practitioners inform pregnant people that an abortion could be a mental health risk, and that a doctor must determine whether a patient was of "sound mental health" before allowing them to terminate a pregnancy. Senator Brenda Council of Omaha, an opponent of the fetal pain ban, noted the inconsistency of senators ruling in one bill that the doctor was the ultimate authority on when a pregnant person can have an abortion, then ruling in another bill that the doctor's opinion of a patient's mental health is superseded by that of the legislature. "I'm disturbed about the absolute blatant disregard of this legislature for the health and well-being of the mother," Council stated during the hearing.[20]

After three rounds of hearings, the unicameral legislature overwhelmingly voted to enact the Pain-Capable Unborn Protection Act on April 13, 2010. Only five senators voted against it—including Council and Conrad. It was signed into law by Governor Dave Heineman later that day. Only one amendment made it through to final passage—a six-month moratorium on the bill to allow both sides to prepare for the likely lawsuit to follow. Most expected Dr. Carhart to challenge the bill both on its constitutional merits and on its obvious targeting of him as a provider. Carhart didn't challenge. Instead, he began to practice at a new clinic in Germantown, Maryland, and considered the idea of performing later abortions in Council Bluffs, Iowa, just across the river from Omaha. The Iowa legislature responded to the news of his possible move by attempting to pass a ban on the opening of any new abortion clinics in the city of Council Bluffs.[21] The bill eventually stalled out as the House fought to turn it into a full twenty-week fetal pain ban. However, by that point Carhart had given up on trying to open a clinic in the state.

In the weeks and months that followed, abortion rights supporters and opponents waited for a challenge to the Nebraska fetal pain ban, assuming that someone somewhere would have a case that would instigate it. None ever came. Instead, the model spread across the US, and by January 1, 2019, twenty-four states had passed versions of a twenty week "fetal pain" ban.

But passing those bans didn't mean that every law went into effect.

In 2012, the state of Arizona was the first to have a bill blocked from going into effect, after placing their own ban at twenty weeks gestation—a full two weeks earlier than the model bill's twenty week post-fertilization. Arizona's ban was challenged by the Center for Reproductive Rights, which called it an unconstitutional ban on abortion prior to viability. The restriction was enjoined and an appeal to the Supreme Court to intervene was rejected in 2014.[22] Idaho also had its twenty-week ban challenged in the courts; the liberal Ninth Circuit enjoined that one as well.[23] The ACLU in Georgia also challenged the state's abortion ban, which passed in 2012. That law was blocked until 2016, when the state supreme court allowed it to be enforced.[24]

However, legal intervention was a rare occurrence. Many of the initial twenty-week bans were passed in states where there were no providers offering abortion that late in gestation to start. Because abortion rights supporters didn't have the standing for a lawsuit, abortion opponents were able to lay the groundwork for claims that the bills must be constitutional since no one was challenging them. Next, abortion opponents fed the bills to states with aggressively conservative circuit benches, knowing that right-wing judges would be far more likely to uphold the bans even if they were constitutionally dubious. Fearing just such an outcome, abortion rights activists failed to challenge bans in states like Texas, Missouri and Ohio, and the ability to obtain abortion even at a point where a fetus was not yet viable shrank state by state by state.

While that was a positive outcome for anti-abortion activists, it still didn't help them achieve their original goal: forcing the Supreme Court to take up a case that could offer a replacement for *Roe's* "viability" standard with a legal argument they believed would be especially appealing to Justice Kennedy. Realizing that the only way to successfully get a challenge would be to ban abortion nationally, activists focused on pushing for a federal twenty week ban in Congress.

The House passed a federal version of the bill in 2013, but because the Senate was under Democratic control the vote was mostly political theater. By 2015 both chambers were under Republican majorities and the ban returned, but this time it was blocked by group of Republican House Members—led by North Carolina Rep. Renee Ellmers—who worried that the very restrictive exception for victims of sexual assault would hurt them with voters. The bill stalled again, and Ellmers paid the price by being primaried out of her seat in 2016.

Republicans knew that even if they were to get a bill through the Senate, Democratic President Barack Obama would certainly veto the final law. Yet GOP strategists were eager to force Democratic senators in red states to vote on the bill in order to use those votes against them later, painting the incumbents as "abortion extremists" during their reelection campaigns. By the time Republican President Donald Trump took the oath of office in January of 2017, the GOP suddenly had wrested control of the entire federal government, holding the White House, both chambers of Congress and ability to reshape the entire judiciary.

By then, the "Pain-Capable Unborn Child Protection Act," the brainchild of an incrementalist wing of the anti-abortion movement, and crafted specifically to woo the centrist sensibilities of moderate Supreme Court Justice Anthony Kennedy, was seven years old and methodically working its way to the highest court in the land—and Congress was better positioned to pass it than ever before.

Then in the summer of 2018, Kennedy surprisingly announced his retirement from the Supreme Court, and suddenly the right no longer needed careful, incrementalist laws to tip the court. Despite almost a decade of planning, the twenty-week ban whimpered into the background and abortion opponents fought over which extremist ban to spotlight next.

2

OHIO

FROM BALLOONS TO BEARS, THE "HEARTBEAT BAN" CAUSES HEARTBURN IN ANTI-ABORTION ACTIVISTS

It all started with balloons on Valentine's Day. The Ohio legislature was about to receive a major delivery, and it wasn't a bouquet of roses, or chocolates. Instead, anti-abortion activist Janet Porter had chosen February 14, 2011 as the day to begin the push for a never before considered bill that, if passed, would virtually eliminate abortion in the Buckeye State.

The concept behind HB 125, commonly known as the "heartbeat bill" or "heartbeat ban" was simple enough: If a person went in to get an abortion and a fetal heartbeat could be detected, that person would not be allowed to have the procedure. To launch the campaign to create one of the strictest anti-abortion bills in the United States, Porter's group, Faith2Action, in conjunction with a variety of other anti-abortion action groups, sent thousands of balloons to the Ohio statehouse as a thank you for those who had sponsored the legislation, and a warning to those who stood in its way. Attached to each balloon was a small card that read "Have A Heart. Pass The Heartbeat Bill.[1]"

The heart-shaped delivery was just the beginning of the puns flying across the statehouse floor. One representative who "fought his way through a sea of balloons to get to the podium" [said] "as much as I don't like balloons, this bill really gets to the heart of the matter!" while Republican bill sponsor Lynn Wachtmann remarked, "After all, Ohio is the 'Heart of it all,' so it's only fitting that we protect our fellow human beings with beating hearts."[2]

Watchmann was the ideal representative to spearhead the heartbeat ban. Referred to among colleagues as "Captain Caveman," he was the nominal head of the "Caveman Caucus," a group of Ohio legislators so conservative that they were mostly ignored by the rest of the party until sweeping gains in the 2010 election gave them numbers and power. Watchman was proud to live up to his "caveman" demeanor. "To me, what it meant was the way that we were willing to keep butting our heads against the wall for what we believed in," he told the *Cleveland Plain Dealer* in January 2011.[3] This stubborn tenacity was just what Janet Porter needed to get her heartbeat bill onto the docket; in spite of the numerous supporters she had for the ban in the legislature, the bill wasn't a hit with the entirety of the anti-abortion movement. Many, in fact, regarded it as a waste of time, effort, resources and most especially, money.

Leading anti-abortion activist and attorney James Bopp, Jr. testified against the bill, arguing that it could provide the US Supreme Court the opportunity to consider abortion restrictions through the lens of equal protection guarantees in the Constitution. "If this view gained even a plurality in a prevailing case, this new legal justification for the right to abortion would be a powerful weapon in the hands of pro-abortion lawyers that would jeopardize all current laws on abortion, such as laws requiring parental involvement for minors, waiting periods, specific informed consent information, and so on," Bopp warned. "A law prohibiting abortion would force Justice Kennedy to vote to strike down the law, giving Justice Ginsberg the opportunity to rewrite the justification for the right to abortion for the Court."[4] The risk, it seemed, was too great for even a grand opponent of choice like Bopp.

Also notably opposed to the ban was Ohio Right to Life, which worried that the bill would either sidetrack other anti-abortion bills that had a greater chance at becoming enacted into law, such as a twenty week "fetal pain" ban and a twenty-four week "viability" ban, or actually become law, get challenged in the courts, make it to the Supreme Court and then be used to reaffirm the right to abortion that *Roe v. Wade* already upheld, making it more difficult to overturn the ruling later on. "Timing is everything," said Mike Gonidakis, then the executive director of Ohio Right to Life. "I don't want to get set back 100 years because we pushed too hard to take down (*Roe v. Wade*)."[5] To Porter, the lack of support from Ohio Right to Life had to be the most disappointing part of pushing the legislation, as she had spent nearly a decade as the legislative director of the group.

Porter wasn't the only one disappointed with Ohio Right to Life's opposition to the bill. The group's former President Linda Theis urged unity on the bill, which she called "an engraved invitation to overturn *Roe*."[6] Dr. Jack Willke, the man best known as the physician behind former Missouri Congressman infamous Todd Akin's belief that rape victims couldn't get pregnant [7]and the founder of Ohio Right to Life, went as far as to resign as a board member due to the group's failure to support the heartbeat ban. Willke quickly became one of the biggest advocates for the bill, putting all of his support and influence behind it.

The bill may have been one of the most heavily opposed abortion restrictions in the legislature, but the efforts to get a vote on it ranged from mildly theatrical to completely over the top. For example, in March 2011, just weeks after the Valentine's Day balloons were sent to politicians, a pair of pregnant women came to the hearings and allowed ultrasounds to be performed on them in order to allow the fetal heart-beats to be heard by committee members. "For the first time in a com-mittee hearing, legislators will be able to see and hear the beating heart of a baby in the womb—just like the ones the Heartbeat Bill will protect," explained Porter.[8] The spectacle itself didn't go very well, as only one of the two "witnesses" was able to provide testimony. The nine-week-old fetus, on the other hand, was "barely audible."[9] Audible heartbeat or not, the bill was passed out of committee by a vote of 12 to 11 on March 30, and was sent to the full house.

It was there that things began to stall, as Ohio Right to Life contin-ued to apply pressure on legislative leaders to kill the bill, advising them that if they passed the ban it would do more harm than good. By May, House Speaker William Batchelder was still trying to find a compromise that would make all of the factions of Ohio's anti-abortion movement happy. "Obviously, we don't want to send a bill out that has caused divi-sion within the right-to-life movement, but by the same token we have to make sure that it doesn't come to the floor in a format that isn't as good as we can do because it will undoubtedly end up in the (US) Sixth Circuit (Court of Appeals)," he explained.[10]

No real compromise was ever found, but the house passed the bill nevertheless. On June 28, 2011, the heartbeat ban officially cleared the first chamber of the Ohio state legislature by a 54 to 43 vote. Overjoyed, supporters waited eagerly for the senate to hear the bill next. However, the senate recessed without taking any action on the bill, saying they would consider it once they returned to session in the fall. Porter prepared for their return with a rally on behalf of the ban, complete with luminaries from the anti-abortion movement and even heart-shaped cookies.[11] By November she became even more proactive, as Faith2Action joined with other supporters to create a new group specifically for the purpose of lobbying for the heartbeat ban. Ohio Prolife Action was formed, joining together members of Faith2Action with the angry ex-members of Ohio Right to Life. Linda Theis became the new group's president, Jack Willke vice president.

One of the new group's first endeavors was to broadcast a commercial asking Ohioans who wanted abortion made illegal to call their senators and demand that they support the heartbeat ban. The ad, which ran on *Fox News*, featured a school bus pulling up to two children at a bus stop. A voiceover says that passing the heartbeat ban will "save the equivalent of a school bus full of children every single day." The ad then cut to the image of a bus full of children, with "The heartbeat bill will save 70 Ohio children every day," at the bottom of the screen, followed by a plea to call politicians and ask them to vote for the bill.

In December, a three-day senate hearing was conducted to discuss the bill, with both supporters and opponents testifying. The opposition argued that the most dangerous aspect of the bill was that it would ban abortion at a point in which many people don't even yet know they are pregnant. Because a heartbeat can be detected in some cases as early as eighteen days after conception, and most pregnant people don't even miss their period until fourteen days post conception, the window for obtaining an abortion would be almost impossible to hit. Dr. Lisa Perriera, MD, MPH, OBGYN and member of Physicians for Reproductive Health and Choice said as much in her testimony:

> This bill is effectively a ban on abortion, since the heartbeat is usually detected between the 5th and 6th week after the last menstrual period, often before a woman even realizes that she is pregnant. Banning abortion has never stopped abortion from happening; it has only made abortion unsafe or more difficult to

obtain. Worldwide 48 percent of abortions are unsafe. As a physician I do not want to go back in time and see unsafe abortion in Ohio."[12]

Perriera, who worked with low-income women in the state through her work at Preterm, an abortion clinic in Cleveland, was especially concerned about the effect that a virtual ban would have on her own patients. "It would have presented a lot of issues. It would have required women to travel to other places to have abortions if they wanted to have them," she said. "But, the patients that I care for are of so little means already, it would have forced them to continue their pregnancy. We would have had a lot more women that are having babies that don't want to have them. It's not a way to bring children into the world."[13]

Kellie Copeland, executive director of NARAL Pro-Choice Ohio, attended the hearings and later reported the impact that the testimony of Perriera and several other physicians had on the committee. "I think one of the other things that got in particular, the chairman of the senate house committee was the number of physicians who came and testified," she recalls. "He asked one of the doctors who is with the Ohio state medical center what would happen if this bill passed, in terms of his colleagues, and I think the doctor really shocked him because he said that doctors who are residents in Ohio now are leaving because of the bills they already passed."

Copeland was referring to four bills which had passed the year before, which banned, among other things, later abortion without a health exception, and insurers from covering abortion in insurance plans. "The chairman physically sat back in his seat," Copeland said. "He was really shocked by that. Every doctor who testified after that, the chairman asked them the same question and they said the same thing. The doctors were leaving the state in droves. It's a bad environment already and the heartbeat bill would make it impossible. Ohio already has an OBGYN shortage, that's pretty commonly known. So to have doctor after doctor testify that, 'If you pass this, we're leaving.' I think it really shook them up. I don't think that's something they expected to hear. They should have, of course."[14]

Although the testimony obviously moved the senators to be cautious about the bill, it was the actions of those who supported the ban that was the final straw. Eager to calm Senate President Tom Niehaus's worries about the bill not being clear enough, backers proposed some adjustments to the bill. Those "adjustments" ended up being twenty proposed amendments. As a result, Niehaus called off the rest of the hearings. "These eleventh hour revisions only serve to create more uncertainty about a very contentious issue," he said. "We've now heard hours of testimony that indicate a sharp disagreement within the pro-life community over the direction of this bill, and I believe our members need additional time to weigh the arguments." The bill was officially tabled until the following year.[15]

•

With no idea of when a vote would be scheduled in the senate, heartbeat ban supporters began 2012 on a mission to get a vote on the bill, and were willing to consider any kind of tactic to make that happen—including the use of children and stuffed animals. In January, Pro-Life Action bused fifty children to the capitol to lobby for a hearing on the Heartbeat Ban. One young boy, only eight years old, chastised the senators, saying, "I'm here to save babies with beating hearts. And I want to tell the senators to pass the Heartbeat Bill right now. And when I mean right now, I mean right now."[16] The children didn't come empty-handed, either, as each one brought along a stuffed bear to give to a senator. The bear came complete with a recorded heartbeat.

Although the event got the attention of the media, the senators were less than impressed. Nearly all of them tried to return their bears, saying they were concerned that the amount the animals cost exceeded the maximum they were allowed to receive in gifts.[17] The bears and children were also seen as manipulative ploys by some senators. "I'm not at all supportive of the bill, and I'm not supportive of them sending kids in my office with a teddy bear that mimics a heartbeat, either," Democratic Senator Shirley Smith told the *Huffington Post*. "I thought that was a very cheap exploitation of kids. I would rather them come in my office and ask to sit down and talk about it, rather than send a kid into my office. I didn't like it at all."[18]

Kellie Copeland also heard from many legislators who were concerned about children being used as pawns in the group's anti-abortion message. "I think a lot of our folks looked at the flowers and other things as stunts. I think that was how it was received in a lot of the Senate offices as well," she said. "The one that got a little different reaction was when they had the children come and lobby and deliver the teddy bears. One of the Senate staffers told me that it kind of disturbed them because some of the kids were quite young. Their family walked them to the door of the Senate office but didn't go in with them. She told me that the kids that walked into her office looked pretty scared and intimidated. So I think that was received with a little more concern, how the kids may have been exploited."[19]

Despite the controversy, the bears—and their young messengers— were just the beginning. On February 14, 2012, one year after beginning their initial legislative push, the heartbeat ban proponents switched deliveries, with Porter and her cohorts sending 2000 roses to the senate—one dozen roses to senate leaders and eight dozen to each member of the committee that would need to pass the bill before it could go to the full body.

"This is the largest rose delivery in Statehouse history," Porter told report-ers. "Last year we had the largest balloon delivery in Statehouse history, but helium balloons aren't allowed in the Senate as it turns out, so we had a delivery of red roses."[20]

A follow-up push to force the senate to vote on the bill came in April, when Willke took out a full-page ad in the *Columbus Dispatch* attacking senate leaders and others he accused of blocking the bill. The ad, which took the form of an open letter from Willke, demanded Ohioans put pres-sure on the politicians, calling it his "dying wish:" (Willke died almost three years later in February of 2015, at age 89.)

> Republican Senators who ran on a pro-life platform have been sitting on the Heartbeat Bill since it passed the Ohio House of Representatives in June of 2011. They will tell you that they have passed several pro-life bills this session; that is true, and we commend them for their regulatory bills. But make no mis-take, when I founded the pro-life movement it wasn't to regulate how abortions would be done, it was to bring the abortion kill-ing to an END . . . Tell the Ohio GOP Senate to pass the stron-gest Heartbeat Bill now—or we will work to replace them with people who will.[21]

Fed up with the pressure, Tom Niehaus sent an "open letter to pro-life supporters" the following month, making it clear he was no longer going to allow Faith2Action and their followers to badger the senate over not bringing the bill up for a vote:

> [T]he leaders of an organization called Faith2Action have made exaggerated and inflammatory statements about the status of

Substitute House Bill 125 without offering a full explanation of the debate that has emerged within the pro-life community. Their claim that we 'lose more than a school bus full of children everyday'; due to a lack of Senate action on the bill is simply false, and I will not continue to allow the organization to question the commitment of my colleagues to ending the scourge of abortion. Ohio Senate Republicans have done more in the past 16 months to advance the protection of unborn children than any previous General Assembly in our state's history.[22]

Neihaus explicitly stated there would be no vote unless advocates could come up with a compromise that would allow the ban to go into effect without a court battle. That announcement should have been the death knell of the heartbeat ban, but it wasn't, as Porter responded to Niehaus's open letter with one of her own:

[M]ake no mistake: this bill was crafted with the Supreme Court in mind. Those who say the bill is 'unconstitutional,' fail to realize that it is *Roe v. Wade* that is unconstitutional and the only way to reverse it is with a challenge. If the few who stand against the Heartbeat bill want a gutted, 'informed consent only' bill, the best thing the Ohio Senate can do is to pass the strongest Heartbeat Bill now. If the naysayers are right and the courts say 'no' to legal protection, the severability clause will ensure that they still get everything they say they want: Informed Consent. Meanwhile, the 'trigger clause' in the bill will restore legal protection to babies with a favorable High Court ruling in the future. There simply is no downside. As a former President of Ohio Right to Life, Jane Grimm said, 'The Heartbeat Bill is a win-win for everyone. Let the judges decide what's Constitutional and let the Senate do what we elected them to do: Protect human life.'[23]

While it might have been easy to write off Porter's bravado as a symptom of her staunchly anti-abortion politics, the truth is that anti-abortion advocates had every reason to feel comfortable litigating controversial abortion issues like this in the state of Ohio, a jurisdiction in which they'd often found significant success. As an example, in June 2004, Ohio passed HB 126, a law that banned the off-label use of mifepristone, an abortion-inducing medication. On the surface, this would seem to have little to do with the heartbeat ban, other than the fact that both laws restrict abortion rights and access. However, the litigation success surrounding the mifepristone ban helps explain why Ohio anti-abortion advocates pushed so hard for the heartbeat ban, despite strong opposition.

HB 126 regulated and restricted the use of mifepristone by mandating that it could only be administered in the exact dosage that was approved by the Food and Drug Administration back in 2000. This was a specific and intentional prohibition of off-label use of the drug, a common medical practice where doctors alter the dosage of a medication based on current medical knowledge and individual patient needs. The law also imposed criminal and administrative penalties on doctors who prescribed mifepristone past forty-nine days of a woman's last menstrual period (LMP). For women with gestational ages through 49 days LMP, HB 126 required an oral dose of 600 mg of mifepristone followed by an oral administration of a lesser dose of misoprostol two days later as dictated by the FDA's original approval in 2000. However, over time, medical practitioners learned that this dosage was approximately three times the amount of mifepristone needed to induce an abortion in many cases. While ingesting 600 mg of mifepristone is considered safe, there was no advantage, nor medical need, to take three times that amount. The increased dosage also added $200 to the price of an abortion, often leaving surgical abortion as a cheaper option. Yet, that was the law in Ohio, and remained so until the FDA updated its own protocols in 2016.

The state's decision to force doctors to ignore their own experience and best practice in order to adhere to an out of date FDA protocol meant not that only were legislators purposefully driving up the cost and inconvenience of a medication abortion, they also managed to coerce a large number of doctors to refuse to provide them all together. "I think it's definitely true that doctors are not offering medical abortions because of the restrictions," Dr. Lisa Perriera said in 2013. "I know personally, when it came to my institution, I intended to get medical abortion on the formulary for the hospital or at least in my private office. I couldn't get it in the formulary."[24]

The outdated protocol also required women to make four separate clinic visits when taking mifepristone, including one for a follow-up ultrasound to confirm termination of the pregnancy. HB 126 mandated this as the legal course of medical treatment for patients, allowing no exceptions of any kind. It was, in effect, a medical protocol frozen in time. "As an evidence-based medical practitioner it is appalling to me that I can't provide medical abortions the way that it's most effective and most cost effective for patients," Perriera said at the time the law was in effect.

Almost immediately after HB 126 was passed in 2004, Planned Parenthood, on behalf of three affiliates in Ohio and Preterm in Cleveland, filed suit, seeking a preliminary injunction and challenging the bill as unconstitutionally vague, unduly burdensome to abortion rights and violating a woman's right to privacy and bodily integrity. On September 22, 2004, US District Court Judge Susan Dlott sided with the Planned Parenthood plaintiffs, issuing a preliminary injunction preventing the law from going into effect. Abortion opponents appealed the decision to the US Sixth Circuit Court of Appeals, which resulted in the injunction being remanded back to the District Court for further proceedings. The Planned Parenthood plaintiffs renewed their motion to have the bill blocked permanently, and in September 2006, the District Court agreed. Following this, the state of Ohio appealed to the Sixth Circuit to have the injunction overturned and challenged the District Court's finding that the law was unconstitutional because it contained no exception for the health of the pregnant person.

Desiring guidance on how to proceed, the Sixth Circuit certified two questions to the Ohio Supreme Court, asking if HB 126 required that physicians who perform abortions using mifepristone do so in compliance with the forty-nine-day gestational limit described in the FDA approval letter, and if doctors using mifepristone must do so in compliance with the treatment protocols and dosage indications described in the drug's final printed labeling. On July 1, 2009, the Ohio Supreme Court handed anti-abortion activists a decisive victory by answering "yes" to both questions, stating that, "provisions of [HB126] are not ambiguous. It allows physicians to provide or prescribe mifepristone to a patient to induce an abortion only if 'the physician provides the RU-486 (mifepristone) . . . in accordance with all provisions of federal law that govern the use of RU-486 (mifepristone) for inducing abortions.'"

Based on this decision, the US Sixth Circuit Court of Appeals remanded the case back to the District Court, vacating the 2006 permanent injunction but leaving the 2004 preliminary injunction in effect. In May 2011, the District Court again sided with the plaintiffs, ruling that the law was unconstitutional. That order was appealed to the Sixth Circuit. In October a divided court upheld the law[25] and in doing so created yet another dangerous restriction on abortion access based on faulty medical evidence and spurious political motives. As a result, most medical providers in the state stopped using mifepristone completely because of the possible criminal liability attached, making medication abortion essentially unavailable in Ohio until the FDA rules were changed.

It was thus no surprise that Faith2Action continued to aggressively pursue a wide-ranging and controversial abortion restriction like the heartbeat ban, as they had years of judicial signals that the high courts of the state were on their side. They no longer needed to worry about precise legislative language since they could get the desired result they wanted without it. If the bill was vague and tied up in litigation, it would still spook providers from offering the challenged service, and if it was not, the case law was already increasingly shifting rightward away from a pregnant person's liberty interests and toward the state's interest in protecting potential life.

•

Janet Porter's tactics grew far more aggressive after her first failure at passing the ban. Gone were the cookies, balloons, roses, children and stuffed animals. Instead, she and her fellow heartbeat ban proponents dug in their heels even harder, targeting lawmakers with newspaper ads, phone calls, emails and mailings. "This is a warning shot across the bow," Porter said in a 2012 press conference, holding up a copy of a newspaper ad. "You see this? Do you like this? Well it's only going to get more hard hitting. It's going to get more frequent. And as I said before, we're just getting started."[26] The legislative session ended on June 15, 2012 without the bill ever coming up for a vote.

But that was by no means the end of the heartbeat ban saga in Ohio. Year after year the ban would return, each time making it a little bit further through the legislative process. In 2016 abortion opponents finally managed to get the ban to the desk of Republican Governor John Kasich—who by that point had already begun his run for the Republican presidential nomination—only to have him veto the bill. Kasich vetoed the ban again in 2018, and a veto override failed by just one vote in the senate. The veto was one of Kasich's final act as governor of Ohio, as he was term-limited out of office in 2018.

On April 11, 2019, Ohio's new governor, Republican Mike DeWine, signed into law the heartbeat ban, a bill that had taken nearly a decade to get from statehouse to the governor's desk. Ohio Right to Life, once the most powerful opponent of the heartbeat ban, was at the center of the legislative push as one of the ban's biggest cheerleaders. Despite her years of dogged advocacy, Janet Porter wasn't even invited to the signing ceremony.

•

During the years that Ohio struggled through the Sisyphisian process of passing and implementing a heartbeat ban, other states had followed suit. In 2013, North Dakota's Republican Governor Jack Dalrymple signed a ban into law. It was enjoined and then found unconstitutional by a lower court in 2015 and never went into effect. Arkansas also passed a heartbeat bill, but took the unusual step of adding that the ban only applied after the twelfth week of pregnancy, hoping they could maneuver around the courts that way. That also failed, and the Supreme Court refused to hear the case when the state appealed its way up the legal ladder. Iowa was next to pass a heartbeat bill, which was blocked by the State Supreme Court in January 2019 as a violation of the state constitution. Iowa's legislature responded by considering the possibility of changing the constitution to say there is no right to an abortion.

None of these failures impeded the enthusiasm of abortion opponents, who continued to propose the bans over and over again. At the start of the 2019 legislative sessions. new bans were introduced in Mississippi, Minnesota, Tennessee, Florida, Georgia, Kentucky, Louisiana, West Virginia, Missouri. By May 2019, three of these states, in addition to Ohio, had signed bans into law, with only Missouri deviating slightly from the script by setting their ban at eight weeks of pregnancy. In Georgia, the state even took an additional step and entered a potential charge of conspiracy into its law, meaning that an overzealous prosecutor could charge a person who left the state or helped someone leave the state and obtain an abortion somewhere else, even if it was legal in the new destination.

With a newly minted conservative majority in the Supreme Court, the right is more convinced than ever that heartbeat bans will be the ultimate weapon in finally overturning *Roe v. Wade*. And even if they can't succeed in overturning *Roe*, but the Supreme Court eventually lets the restrictions stand, abortion opponents will have essentially banned abortion in many states anyway.

3

THE END OF MEDICATION ABORTION?

IT ALL STARTED IN WISCONSIN

On April 5, 2012, the day before Good Friday, with lawmakers, reporters and policy trackers getting ready for the coming Easter weekend, then Governor Scott Walker quietly signed into law a piece of legislation that would end all medication abortions in the state of Wisconsin.

The Republican governor wasn't normally this shy about his political actions. Within a matter of weeks after being sworn into office in 2011, for example, he began an outright assault on the state's unions, trying to end their power to bargain collectively. Walker's previous efforts to overturn legislation that provided access to reproductive health care and affordable contraceptive coverage had also been done with gusto. The governor, who had been endorsed when he was running for office by both Wisconsin Right for Life and their more rigid, anti-birth control compatriot, Pro-Life Wisconsin, was quite open about his desire to deliver major financial blows to programs that assisted people in obtaining birth control reproductive health services. His 2011 budget eliminated a law that required insurance companies to include birth control in their coverage, declaring it an "unacceptable government mandate on employers with moral objections to these services" which "increases the cost of health insurance for all payers."[1] Walker's 2011 budget also eliminated most of the family planning and preventative health care funds in the BadgerCare program, which offered assistance to low income and uninsured Wisconsinites. The cuts left over 50,000 Wisconsin residents without access to health screenings and preventative care that was projected to save the state $140 million a year in additional medical costs. Walker considered this a necessary tradeoff in order to prevent money from going to Planned Parenthood clinics in Wisconsin.[2]

However, when it came to 2011 Wisconsin Act 217, the "Coercive and Webcam Abortion Prevention Act," Walker couldn't have been more secretive if he had signed the bill into law on Good Friday itself. In fact, that was the day he finally announced to the public that he had signed the Act—along with fifty other bills that he had signed in the previous two days. His spokesperson claimed this wasn't an attempt to hide the legislation, but that it was "simpler" to announce all of the bills at the same time.[3] Many didn't believe that argument, however. "Perhaps he thought that in doing this behind closed doors, with no public notice, before a holiday weekend for many families, his actions would go unnoticed. He was wrong," one Democratic Representative said in a public statement. "We will not be silent—these issues are too important to ignore."[4]

The goal of the "Coercive and Webcam Abortion Prevention Act," which was backed heavily by Wisconsin Right to Life, was to ban "telemed" abortions, a new type of medical access to abortion that was being tried in states across the country. As the ability to see abortion providers was being cut off due to the closing of clinics, long wait periods, regulation of who was allowed to perform procedures and "informed consent" processes like ultrasounds and counseling, it was becoming more difficult for women, especially those in rural areas, to obtain a legal termination. The solution to these myriad problems was telemed abortions. First introduced in 2008 in

Iowa by Planned Parenthood of the Heartland, telemed abortions allowed a patient to go to any of sixteen clinics in the state to speak with a doctor and obtain RU-486, the drug used in medication abortions, but didn't require that patient to travel specifically to the clinic that the doctor worked out of.[5] Dr. Vanessa Cullins, Vice President for Medical Affairs, Planned Parenthood Federation of America, explained the process on *NPR*:

> A woman who generally is in a rural setting or setting where there is very limited physician access, will visit a health care center and meet with a Planned Parenthood of Heartland nurse practitioner. That nurse practitioner who is highly skilled and qualified to provide reproductive and sexual health care will perform both the history, a sonogram will be done and the physical exam . . . The physician will meet the woman through secure Internet-based video conferencing, two-way live conferencing. And it is through this modality that the woman is able to have any questions that she has about the process answered. She can inquire of possible side effects and what to expect as it relates to the medication abortion process. And at the same time, the physician is able to confirm that this woman is indeed a candidate for medication abortion . . . She is receiving high quality, expert care. There's absolutely no evidence that provision of medication abortion through telemedicine is any way dangerous. In fact, the record of Planned Parenthood of Heartland is not only that it is highly safe and effective, but women are highly satisfied with abortion being provided through telemedicine services.[6]

Patients may have been satisfied with the procedure, but abortion opponents were appalled once they recognized the potential it had to expand access to abortion. Troy Newman, the president of Operation

Rescue, one of the country's most adamant and vitriolic anti-abortion organizations, filed a complaint in 2010 with the Iowa State Board of Medicine alleging that telemed abortions were unlawful because the woman didn't meet face to face with a doctor, so there wasn't a "licensed physician" providing the abortion. "This is a prescription for disaster," Newman told the *New York Times.* "You are removing the doctor-patient relationship from this process. And think about it: With this scheme, one abortionist sitting in his pajamas at home could literally do thousands of abortions a week. This is about expanding their abortion base . . . One way or another, we're going to shut this scheme down," he promised. "Health care just isn't a one-size-fits-all package of pills. And yet there it is—prearranged, prepackaged, out pops that package of pills—pop!"[7]

While Operation Rescue and other anti-abortion organizations tried to end telemed abortions by going to the Iowa Board of Medicine, lawmakers in the state who opposed the practice took a different approach—a funding ban. Though Planned Parenthood insisted that no federal money had been used for telemed abortions, abortion opponents refused to believe them. During the 2011 debate over HR 2112, the Agriculture Appropriations bill, Iowa Republican Congressman Steve King tacked on an amendment that would ban Planned Parenthood from receiving any sort of federal funding for telemedicine programs in general, even if the funding was to support its own infrastructure to perform other medical practices remotely. According to King, those funds could be inadvertently used for "robo-skype" abortions. "Some [sic] of us signed a letter—70 of us—to Kathleen Sebelius and asked if they had distributed grants for telemedicine to any of the abortion providers including Planned Parenthood," King told *Lifenews.* "There [sic] response came back in the affirmative that they had issued several grants to Planned Parenthood. And these funds, as near as we can determine, are being used to provide telemedicine for the robo-abortions, the robo-Skype abortions [sic] as I've described."[8] Despite the support of the amendment in the US Senate by then Republican Minority Leader Jim DeMint, the proposal did not pass.

In May 2012, King tried again, this time soliciting co-sponsors for what he called the "Telemedicine Safety Act," a bill that was supposed to ensure that no federal money was used to support telemed abortion services. According to the bill

(a) No funds made available under a telemedicine law... may be used for telemedicine abortions or for assistance to facilities that offer telemedicine abortions.

(b) No equipment, infrastructure, or other items purchased using funds made available under a telemedicine law may be used for telemedicine abortions.[9]

This was, in essence, a standalone version of the amendment that had been tacked onto the agriculture bill the year before, but without any pressing matter attached to it, the bill stalled out in committee. By this time, though, it was no longer necessary for anti-abortion activist to try and defund telemed abortions, as the process had actually become more useful to the movement as a tool to advocate for new restrictions on RU-486.

Legislating medication abortions wasn't a totally new concept, as Ohio already had passed its own bill in 2004 that mandated how to provide RU-486 based on FDA regulations versus medical best practices. But that lone restriction was it, until anti-abortion politicians started embracing the idea of legislating non-surgical abortions out of existence. "[W]e just did not see [medication abortion restrictions] up until 2011," said Elizabeth Nash of the Guttmacher Institute. "Medication abortion was approved in 2000 and for the most part, we didn't see anything on that method until 2011 and, all of a sudden, we see these bills, and they become law, whether it be a telemedicine ban or an FDA protocol bill . . . These things essentially stop providers from administering medication abortion, either because you're using an outdated protocol that nobody would use . . . Or you're doing this telemedicine ban which you wouldn't think would shut down clinics but it shut down every clinic or it shut down the use of medication abortion completely in Wisconsin. I just think you adopt those kinds of restrictions and you are not chipping away at *Roe*, you are hacking away at *Roe* without ever entering a courtroom."[10] With the "Coercive and Webcam Abortion Prevention Act," Wisconsin lawmakers could proactively ban telemed abortions while putting more pressure—as well as potential penalties—on any doctor who performed a medication abortion in the state, even if the doctor provided the pills in person.

Wisconsin Right to Life put the full force of its lobbying arm behind Act 217, encouraging supporters to sign petitions, contact legislators, and to fill the hearing room when the bill was introduced in the House committee. The group also promoted a video of a "Dramatized RU-486 Chemical Abortion Interview" reenactment meant to explain why women needed to meet multiple times with the same doctor prior to termination. In the video, a doctor tells a woman who is uncertain as to whether or not she should have an abortion that once it is clear she doesn't have an ectopic pregnancy, she can begin the procedure. "After all, it's just tissue," the women tells the doctor, obviously trying to convince herself that she is justified in ending the pregnancy. "Well, we are all 'just tissue,'" the doctor replies, as the camera goes shaky and the picture flickers in and out. The doctor then begins to describe the procedure, including "cutting off nutrient to the embryo" to kill it, as well as the physical and emotional pain the woman will experience in the "several weeks" it could take to fully complete the abortion. "The pain while you are waiting for it to happen may be hard. Cleaning up afterwards may be harder," the doctor says dispassionately. "Participating in your own abortion may be the hardest part of all. Are you prepared for what you are going to see and experience?" The woman responds that she "hadn't really thought about that," looking away from the camera, near tears. The video ends with her sitting in her car, watching a mother carry a young toddler to a nearby vehicle.[11]

Whether the over the top advocacy worked, or the bill was a already a sure thing in the Republican-dominated Assembly, Act 217 passed during a knock-down, drag out legislative session that went far into the night. (The debate lasted nearly three hours and included a Democratic attempt to add an amendment forcing men to have rectal exams prior to receiving erectile dysfunction drugs.)[12] Having previously passed the state senate, the bill went straight to the governor for signature on March 16, 2012. Despite the vast support of the legislature and his outspoken opposition to the right to choose, Governor Walker waited several weeks before signing Act 217 into law. Why would a man who had made restricting access to abortion, subsidized birth control, family planning, and even emergency contraception the center point of his election campaign in 2010 try to hide one of the most sweeping abortion restriction bills the state of Wisconsin had ever seen? It could have been an attempt to rehabilitate his image as he grew closer to a pending recall election that would have evicted him from office before he had even finished his first term. No governor prior to Walker had ever successfully weathered a recall effort, and the conservative politician might have felt that the last thing he needed was to appear to be doing a victory lap in another battle in the war against women.

Still, there was a more likely reason for his silence: it gave his opponents less time to marshal their resources against the bill. As news of Act 217 being signed into law began to trickle out into the media on Good Friday 2012, many of those against the bill had already left for the long weekend, planning to resume their push the following week to call on the governor to veto the legislation. With the law scheduled to go into effect on April 20, two weeks from the point in which Walker had signed the bill, by the time medical personnel and advocates were back in their offices the following week, several days would have already passed. That provided a much smaller window of time for those groups who provided medication abortions to talk to their legal counsels and come up with a game plan to continue providing services under the new law.

The most common set of drugs used in a medication abortion are mifepristone, i.e., RU-486, and misoprostol. Mifepristone blocks the body's production of progesterone, a necessary hormone for continuing a pregnancy, allowing the lining of the uterus to thin and the cervix to soften. Given later on, misoprostol causes contractions, which allows the body to release the contents of the uterus, including the lining, embryo or fetus, placenta and any other products of conception that remain. There are a number of advantages to a medication abortion over a surgical one, ranging from time spent in the doctor's office, the ability to abort in privacy, the less invasive nature of the procedure, and the amount of recovery time needed.

In a typical medication abortion in a state like Wisconsin—which also has a 24-hour mandatory waiting period—a person seeking a termination meets with a doctor who discusses the procedure. The patient can then return to the clinic after the 24 hours has passed, when they would then be able to take mifepristone. The patient would also be given misoprostol to take later on, but is allowed to leave the clinic in order to be at home or wherever they choose when the abortion occurs. After the abortion is finished, the patient is encouraged to schedule an appointment in the clinic or to see their primary care physician or other doctor for follow up care, including determining if the abortion is fully complete.

These guidelines, which had been developed and endorsed as best practices by medical professionals, were not good enough for the legislators who wrote the "Coercive and Webcam Abortion Prevention Act." Instead, under the Act, pregnant people had to meet in person with the same doctor multiple times throughout the course of an abortion, starting first with the intake, then again when they obtain the mifepristone and then again 12 to 18 days after the drug was taken.

A major difficulty of complying with Act 217 was the doctor's responsibility to follow up with the patient when it came to post-procedure appointments. Based on the legislation, though the patient was allowed to refuse a follow up appointment, the doctor could still be held responsible for not seeing that patient, which could result in professional discipline and even a potential loss of his or her medical license. The doctor was also now held responsible for screening a patient for potential "coercion," a sign that the decision to abort was not being brought about through outside pressure through a family member or partner. The onus would be on the doctor if a patient returned later and said that the decision was coerced, and the physician could be sued. Act 217 created a new level of legislative interference in medical protocol, creating criminal penalties for doctors who were simply following medical best practices and individual patient circumstances. Doctors who broke the new law could potentially be charged with a Class I felony, resulting in a $10,000 fine, a three-and-a half-year prison sentence, or both.[13]

That doctors could be convicted of felonies was a valid fear for medical practitioners, who almost unanimously called on Walker to veto Act 217. The Medical College of Wisconsin, Wisconsin Medical Society and the Wisconsin Academy of Family Physicians all opposed the bill, an unprecedented move from organizations that normally avoided endorsing or opposing legislation, in order to appear non-political.[14] According to Dr. Fredrik Broekhuizen, a Wisconsin member of the board of Physicians for

Reproductive Health and Choice, it was the first time that the Wisconsin Medical Society had taken a stand on any abortion law.[15] Multiple advocacy groups also stated that the law was too vaguely written to be certain what would and wouldn't be enforced. Dr. Broekhuizen believed the bill was meant to present a set of "minimum safety standards" for patient care that would go mostly under the radar, allowing an "overzealous prosecutor" to later charge a doctor based on one of the vague, legally-ambiguous points in the law, putting medical abortion availability for the entire state at risk.

If that was indeed the plan, it would leave doctors holding the bag. By writing a bill that would make any failure to follow every step in the bill a felony, a doctor who was charged with breaking the law would be unable to defend themselves in court without assuming enormous legal bills. Although doctors have insurance that pays for their defense in a malpractice suit, there is no such coverage when it comes to defending from a felony, since most professional liability policies contain "crime/fraud" exceptions. "What we do would be 'defensible,'" said Dr. Broehhuizen. "But we'd have to pay to defend it."[16]

Because of the nebulous legal terrain that Act 217 created, Planned Parenthood of Wisconsin announced on April 21, 2012 that until their lawyers could better determine the ramifications of the bill, medication abortions at all their clinics would be suspended. The news was shocking. Planned Parenthood owned all but one of the abortion clinics in the state in 2012, and roughly 25 percent of women who came in for the procedure opted for a medication abortion.

Nicole Safar, the group's public policy director, noted that with Governor Scott Walker signing the bill into law over a holiday weekend, their lawyers simply have not had enough time to fully analyze the impact the new law had on the procedure and how, or even if, their providers could comply without endangering their own careers. "We have our lawyers looking at ambiguity," explained Safar. "We have not even had two weeks to look at this. The legislature is actually dictating patient care, and we are working with our lawyers to see how this effects medical best practices and procedures." She said it was "too risky" to perform the procedure in the state until the law was straightened out.[17] Abortion opponents were joyous, as they had found a way to further restrict abortion access in Wisconsin. Barbara Lyons, Executive Director of Wisconsin Right to Life, called the news a "true victory for Wisconsin women." "[B]ecause chemical abortions comprise 26% of Wisconsin abortions," she said, "their suspension will result in another decline in Wisconsin abortions which is great news for mothers and babies."[18] Pro-Life Wisconsin was more cautious, concerned that the Planned Parenthood move was just a ploy to convince anti-abortion activists to let down their guard. While they publicly told a local news station, "Any day Planned Parenthood is not performing an RU-486 abortion is a good one," on their own website, they added this caveat: "However, we remain suspicious of their plans."[19]

On May 11, 2012, three weeks after the Planned Parenthood announcement, Affiliated Medical Services, the last provider of medication abortions in the state of Wisconsin, announced on its website that it would no longer offer the service either. Less than a month after Walker had signed Act 217 into law, access to medication abortions in the state of Wisconsin was gone. NARAL Pro-Choice Wisconsin lamented the loss of access in the state. "It is unacceptable that women are losing health care options because Walker has put his extreme social agenda ahead of what is best for women's health," Lisa Subeck, the group's executive director, told reporters. "Women lose out when out of control politicians like Scott Walker practice medicine without a license and interfere in the relationship between doctors and their patients."[20]

On Tuesday, December 11, 2012, almost eight months after announcing they would no longer provide medication abortions in the state, Planned Parenthood of Wisconsin announced it had filed suit against the enforcement of Act 217, claiming that Act 217 unconstitutionally violated due process as it was too vague in explaining what doctors must do to satisfy the components of the bill. Lawyers for the group said that the organization waited months to file suit in order to determine if there was any way that they could potentially comply with the new law but simply couldn't find a way to do so without opening their doctors up to possible legal issues. "Planned Parenthood wanted to comply. They did not take the decision to litigate lightly," Susan Crawford, Senior Associate, Cullen, Weston, Pines and Bach told reporters during a conference call announcing the suit. "The process takes time, it is a huge use of resources. It was not brought about lightly and only after great consideration."[21] "The very personal opinion of how to terminate a pregnancy is taken away from women," added Teri Huyck, then the President and CEO of Planned Parenthood of Wisconsin. "We are in court to make sure that once again pregnancy decisions reside with the woman her family and her faith, with the counsel of her doctor."[22]

Medication abortion remained completely unavailable for over a year in the state of Wisconsin, and didn't return until June of 2013. At that point Planned Parenthood announced they would once again be offering the service, saying they had figured out how to adhere to all of the onerous and medically unnecessary rules without jeopardizing patient care or putting their doctors in danger of a lawsuit.

•

With Act 217, anti-abortion advocates in Wisconsin were able to build on the lessons they had learned from their colleagues in Ohio, showing how a purposefully vague anti-abortion statute could successfully eradicate access while simultaneously creating fodder for a legal challenge to *Roe v. Wade*. There were actually several aspects of Act 217 that were designed to make specific inroads against *Roe* and to further segregate out the delivery of reproductive health care. First was the idea of "coercion" in the context of informed consent. Historically, dictating medical procedures or patient disclosures under the guise of "empowering" the patient with information so they can properly consent to the procedure have been the most successful means of restricting abortion access. However, informed consent for medical treatment is a legal concept grounded in notions of fundamental human rights, a fact Act 217 and other similar bills that attempt to tackle the idea of "coerced abortions" blithely overlook. Informed consent requirements "must be calculated to inform the woman's free choice, not hinder it,"[23] and because an informed consent requirement must "facilitate[] the wise exercise" of a person's right to abortion, such a requirement presents an undue burden unless it provides "truthful and not misleading" information.[24] In many ways, anti-coercion bills are the colonization of the idea of informed consent. Built into the idea of informed consent is the presumption that such consent is given voluntarily. Coercion bills take that idea, turn it on its head and shift the legal burden in establishing voluntary consent to physicians. For example, the language of Wisconsin Section 253.10(3)(b), the state's "coercion" bill reads:

> Voluntary consent. Consent under this section to an abortion is voluntary only if the consent is given freely and without coercion by any person. The physician who is to perform or induce the abortion shall determine whether the woman's consent is, in fact, voluntary. Notwithstanding par. (c) 3., the physician shall make the determination by speaking to the woman in person, out of the presence of anyone other than a person working for or

with the physician. If the physician has reason to suspect that the woman is in danger of being physically harmed by anyone who is coercing the woman to consent to an abortion against her will, the physician shall inform the woman of services for victims or individuals at risk of domestic abuse and provide her with private access to a telephone.

Other than taking the pregnant person outside the presence of others and asking if they are being coerced into terminating a pregnancy, the law gives zero guidance on how doctors are to make such a determination, let alone prove it later should it be challenged. Furthermore, doctors are already mandatory reporters, so should a patient present with evidence of assault or domestic violence, physician's standard of care already dictates they make a reasonable inquiry into that suspicion.

Finally, any informed consent requirement in the context of abortion regulation must also consider the doctor's constitutional speech rights as well. In *Casey*, the Supreme Court held that "a requirement that a doctor give a woman certain information as part of obtaining her consent to an abortion" implicates a physician's First Amendment right not to speak, "but only as part of the practice of medicine, subject to reasonable licensing and regulation by the State."[25] Normally, the government's ability to restrict speech is limited, but in the context of abortion disclosures, that is not quite so. But because states regulate the practice of medicine, and do so to provide a common good for all, the court held in *Casey*, doctors' First Amendment rights could be restricted, and as it turns out, even circumscribed. So the question remains, was it reasonable for the state of Wisconsin to mandate an additional, nebulous procedure in the course of treatment of a person seeking an abortion and attach criminal penalties for failing to comply?

The other issue waiting to surface in the wake of Act 217 is the manner in which it restricts the use of RU-486. According to *Gonzales v. Cahart*, states are free to regulate specific medical practices, even if those regulations are not grounded in medical consensus. The requirements that patients follow-up multiple times with the proscribing doctors fly in the face of the scientific evidence that RU-486 is as safe and effective as a surgical abortion when done within the first nine weeks of pregnancy.[26] Furthermore, in a state as rural as Wisconsin, telemed abortions represent a real benefit for many women who are isolated from urban health clinics or hospitals where alternative abortion care could be available if needed. For these women, Act 217 literally cut off access to the safest, cheapest and most immediate abortion care and instead exposed them to greater risk and expense.

•

Unlike so many other abortion restrictions introduced around this time period, Wisconsin's Act 217 didn't open up the door to copycat legislation. Instead, several states tested out a wide variety of tactics for restricting or eliminating the ability to obtain medication abortion, with a special focus on targeting telemed abortion programs, like the one in Iowa, before they could be replicated in other states. Eventually, the "Abortion Inducing Drugs Safety Act," model legislation crafted by Americans United for Life became the most popular bill, forcing pregnant patients to be in the physical presence of a doctor in order to begin the medication process. As of 2019, seventeen states had these "telemed abortion ban" laws in effect, thereby blocking what had the potential to be the biggest and most effective expansion of abortion access since *Roe* was settled.[27]

In Iowa, Republican Governor Terry Branstad replaced members of the Iowa State Board of Health with abortion opponents over the years, and in 2013 the board shut down the entire state telemed program, calling it "an unsafe medical practice" despite the fact that no patient had ever filed a complaint. In 2015, the Iowa Supreme Court ruled against the board, but by that point the damage was irreversible.[28] Between the state's continuous abortion restrictions and ongoing attempts to strip funding from Iowa's Planned Parenthood affiliate, rural clinics were already closing, decreasing the number of places left to even participate in the program. Another round of state defunding in 2017 escalated the process, and by the end of 2018 only eight clinics remained—five of which offered medication abortion.[29]

By 2019, telemed abortion programs were slowly expanding again, despite the attacks from anti-abortion forces, but unsurprisingly were restricted primarily to states that already had fairly good abortion access to start. Medication abortions could be legally obtained via mail in Hawaii, Oregon, Washington State, Maine and New York through a pilot program run by Gynuity Health Projects,[30] or via telemed through a program that Planned Parenthood announced in 2018 that would invest in expanding access to multiple states across the nation.[31]

Of course, mediation abortion could also be obtained outside an approved legal clinic setting, and the number of people reaching out to these sources continued to grow. The question then became what would happen when a person was caught, and how willing the right-wing was to jail that pregnant person as a result? That answer? Far more willing than you could imagine.

4

IDAHO

JAILING THE "MOTHER"

Jennie Linn McCormack believed that having an abortion was the best mothering decision she could make for her children. Like a vast percentage of the one in three women who get an abortion, McCormack already was a mother. Her three children, one of whom was still a toddler, already stretched her thin both financially and emotionally. The man who had gotten her pregnant was in jail. Adding another child to the family simply wasn't something she could do without neglecting the children she had already dedicated her life to.

McCormack knew that getting an abortion was not going to be easy. She lived in Bannock County, a rural, heavily Mormon part of Idaho, and finding a local provider who could do a termination was impossible. So was traveling over two hours by car to Salt Lake City, Utah, the site of the closest abortion clinic. McCormack didn't have a car of her own, and with a twenty-four mandatory waiting period in Utah (this was in 2010; currently the waiting period in Utah is three days), she would need to either make the trip twice or stay overnight and pay for the cost of a hotel.

This was on top of paying for the actual abortion, which was no small cost itself, since McCormack believed she was in her second trimester, a point in which the price of an abortion begins to escalate significantly.

In desperation, McCormack spoke to her sister, who ordered RU-486 off the internet and had the pills shipped to her. McCormack just wanted to quickly and privately end her pregnancy and move on with trying to make the best life she could for her children with the meager resources she had. However, her private medical procedure didn't stay so "private." Instead, when McCormack miscarried after taking RU-486, she realized that she had been quite wrong about how far along she was, and that the fetus was more developed than a fourteen-week pregnancy should have been. In a panic, she wrapped up the body and placed it in a shoebox. A few days later she moved the box to a covered grill on her front porch as she tried to decide what to do next. She confided her dilemma to a close friend, not expecting that her friend would tell his sister what had happened. The man's sister informed the police, who went to McCormack's house and arrested her for "unlawful abortion." "There's other things she could have done," the informant, Brenda Carnahan, told the *Associated Press*. "She could have asked for some type of help."[1] Carnahan believed that it was her responsibility to speak for the baby. "I'm a grandmother myself. And the love and the compassion I have for my grandkids? They're my life. And I felt that if somebody didn't speak up for this baby, who would? It doesn't have a voice anymore."[2]

McCormack was arrested under a 1972 statute that made it illegal in the state of Idaho to terminate a pregnancy unless you were a physician, and only allowed abortions past the first trimester to be performed in a hospital setting. Since the law was nearly forty years old at the time of McCormack's abortion in December 2010, it was difficult to be certain if the statute applied to procuring drugs off the internet. However, Bannock

County prosecuting attorney Mark L. Hiedeman decided that any abortion initiated by a non-Idaho practicing doctor fell under the terms of the "unlawful abortion" statute, and as a result, McCormack was charged with a felony for ending the pregnancy on her own, outside of a hospital. "It just felt like it fit the statute . . ." Hiedeman said. "[And] this wasn't the first time this has happened. She's had abortions before, and miscarriages. I mean, she was obviously getting pregnant time and time again and not protecting the unborn fetus."[3] Hiedeman's comments made it seem as if he was looking for a way to punish McCormack for her personal life, and what he saw as a woman using abortion as a form of birth control.

Ultimately, the county's attempt to convict McCormack failed. With Idaho attorney (and licensed physician) Rick Hearn acting as her defense lawyer, the case against McCormack was dismissed due to lack of corroborating evidence that a crime had been committed.[4] There was no packaging from the abortion drug lying around her house, no sign of RU-486 in the fetus (medications that induce abortions cannot be seen in any blood tests, either in the system of the patient or the miscarried fetus or embryo), and nothing that could prove that McCormack did in fact take the medication or that it resulted in her miscarriage. Despite this, the judge still left the case open for the prosecution to re-file should new evidence be found. McCormack, unwilling to live her life with the specter of prison looming over her, decided with the help of her lawyer to sue the state instead, challenging several abortion restrictions, including the "fetal pain" restriction on abortions after twenty weeks and the "illegal abortion" statute, seeking to have them both declared unconstitutional. This would be the first challenge to the so-called "fetal pain" bans that had started spreading across the country in the wake of Nebraska's first successful passage of one in 2010.

McCormack and Hearn initially succeeded in obtaining an injunction that prohibited any future criminal prosecutions under the state's illegal abortion law. Challenging the twenty-week abortion ban was less simple. When McCormack filed her lawsuit, she was no longer pregnant. Her alleged abortion had happened on December 24, 2010, but the twenty-week fetal pain ban in the state of Idaho didn't go into effect until January 1, 2011. Since McCormack wasn't pregnant when the law went into effect, she technically didn't have standing to challenge it, the state argued, despite the fact that she was arrested and charged after the law went into effect. The court agreed, but would not dismiss McCormack's suit until the standing issue was resolved on appeal. This left the immediate challenge tied up in appellate review before the constitutionality of the law would even begin to be addressed. If there was no other plaintiff to challenge the law, the likelihood of the original injunction being lifted and the law being implemented dramatically increased. In effect, this meant that Idaho's twenty-week fetal pain ban and illegal abortion statute would remain as the law of the land.

While McCormack may have lacked standing to challenge the abortion laws according to the lower court, Rick Hearn didn't have that problem. In an unprecedented move, he filed a motion to intervene in the case, making him a party to the same lawsuit he was pursuing on behalf of McCormack. His argument was that, as a licensed physician, he might have need at some future date to perform an abortion past the arbitrary, pre-viability timeline established by the state. "The judge on two occasions had found Jennie lacked the standing to bring her case challenging the laws that burdened doctors in performing abortions," Hearn said, explaining why he inserted himself into what was originally a suit meant to protect pregnant people from being arrested for obtaining abortions. "The court had found that Jennie did have standing for any laws that she would be punished under or would be put in jail for, but declined to find that she had standing and therefore it had jurisdiction to reach issues under those same laws as applied to the providers."[5]

The Supreme Court gave doctors standing to file suit against abortion regulations in 1976, in *Singleton v. Wulff*.[6] In that case, two Missouri abortion doctors filed suit against the state's welfare statute because it would not grant benefits for abortions that were not considered to be medically necessary. The case turned on the question of who could best represent the interests of patients seeking an abortion when those patients could not represent those interests themselves.[7] Based on the decision in the *Wulff* case, the answer was physicians. According to the ruling, "[a] woman cannot safely secure an abortion without the aid of a physician, and an impecunious woman cannot easily secure an abortion without the physician being paid by the State."[8] Therefore, the Court concluded, a pregnant person could only exercise the right to choose an abortion with the aid of a doctor. Thus, doctors should have standing to challenge any abortion restrictions themselves.[9]

As a practitioner in Idaho, Rick Hearn had an immediate interest in challenging the strict abortions laws of the state, as he was potentially the only provider many women would have access to. "As a physician I am obviously such a provider, and so I was able to correct that problem by intervening to challenge the laws because those laws can be used to punish me," Hearn said. "The court did find that I had standing to do that."

Hearn had standing for a second reason as well. "While I have to be injured by the threat of being prosecuted, it is not my right to perform abortions. I don't have any constitutional right to practice medicine, much less to perform an abortion. So I will not be asserting any rights that I have. And the courts have already found that doctors can assert the rights of their patients in the abortion context. So a doctor, or a group of doctors and providers, does have standing to represent the rights of their patient."

Although Hearn hadn't practiced medicine in several years, his motion to intervene was granted, making him a plaintiff in the lawsuit he had started on McCormack's behalf.[10] Yet while Hearn was able to represent her interests to some degree, in reality, the court had largely removed McCormack from the proceedings and placed her interests in the hands of surrogates. In a sense, the court had determined that everyone but McCormack had an interest in challenging abortion laws in the state of Idaho. Hearn summed it up like this, "It appears to me to be paternalistic to say that women must depend upon primarily male doctors to get into court to assert their rights." In some ways, this was a logical extension of women's historical legal status under common law, where they used to be considered akin to juveniles or other wards of the state. This lack of legal capacity has helped foster the belief that the state has an obligation to protect them, especially in the case of abortion.[11]

By recognizing abortion rights in *Roe v. Wade*, the Supreme Court also recognized the legal interests of third parties to have a say in the termination of a pregnancy. In some instances, such as with Hearn, the interests of these third-parties advocates align with those of the patient seeking an abortion, but more often than not, the situation is murkier. Adding an additional layer of consent has long been a ploy abortion opponents have used to limit a person's right to an abortion, with varying levels of success. Consent issues first came up in 1976 in *Planned Parenthood v. Danforth*, which challenged a pair of abortion requirements in the state of Missouri: one, that a married woman seeking an abortion had to get her husband's written consent first; and two, that a pregnant minor under the age of eighteen who is not emancipated must have a parent's written consent before being able to terminate a pregnancy.[12] In both instances, the state's inference was clear—a pregnant spouse or teen was not considered capable of making a decision on her own, and needed to confer with and gain permission from someone else in either a direct or implied paternal sense of the word.

Though both requirements for consent were ultimately found unconstitutional in *Danforth*, that didn't stop abortion foes from continuing to use consent as a means of coercing pregnant women, and in particular teens, into giving birth. Indeed, if the state had an interest in protecting potential life thanks to *Casey*, then, according to anti-abortion activists, that interest only increased when it came to juvenile pregnancy. For example, in July 2011, the Pennsylvania Pastor's Network lent its support to a pregnant fourteen-year-old who was being pressured by her mother to have an abortion. The girl eventually won an injunction against her mother with assistance from the Independence Law Center in Pennsylvania, who argued that it was illegal to coerce a minor into having an abortion.[13] The Pastor's Network applauded the girl's decision to make a choice independent of her parent's wishes, saying, "This is a hard road ahead for this young girl, but we applaud her and the future paternal grandparents of the child for standing up for life. Although this girl is in a difficult situation today, it is a blessing that she has chosen not to make a mistake that would end a child's life."[14] Ironically, the same Independence Law Center had earlier argued for stricter rulings for judges who allowed parental consent bypasses so minors could obtain abortions, saying judges needed to do more to "respect parental authority."[15]

Much like physician intervention rights, parental consent and judicial bypass rest largely on the argument that the decision to terminate a pregnancy impacts the interests of other parties, who should then have a say in the matter.[16] In no other area of the law does an issue that is so intimate get decided by committee. As of February 2019, thirty-seven states required some form of parental consent or notification in order for a pregnant minor to obtain an abortion, all with varying availability for judicial bypass. And, like access to abortion itself, judicial bypass is also being targeted by abortion opponents who want stricter rules on which judges can offer a bypass, such as requiring teens to only use a judge in their current town to stop so-called "district shopping" to find more sympathetic judges, or allowing judges to take their time in making a decision, adding days or longer on top of specific waiting periods in clinics prior to the procedure.

•

Unlike parental consent, spousal consent laws have generally been a less effective means of limiting a woman's right to choose. The proposition of spousal consent was one of the issues that brought about the challenge that became *Planned Parenthood v. Casey*, and following that decision, few on the anti-abortion side seemed anxious to push those restrictions again. Ohio State Representative John Adams proposed a bill in 2007, but it went nowhere, as did a 2010 version[17] Missouri lawmaker Rick Brattin tried one in 2014, but his attempts also faltered. But while actual spousal consent bills wither in committees, the paternalistic assumption that a pregnant person doesn't have the autonomy to make their own decision on abortion has manifested in the proliferation of "informed consent" paperwork and prepared scripts that doctors in many states must offer women seeking abortions, which are ironically dubbed "A Woman's Right To Know."

But while direct consent was a failure, spouses and partners gained power in other ways. In 2012, the "Pain-Capable Unborn Child Protection Act" stated that "A qualified plaintiff may in a civil action obtain injunctive relief to prevent an abortion provider from performing or attempting further abortion . . ." According to the law, a "qualified plaintiff" is defined as "a woman upon whom an abortion is performed" or "any person who is the spouse, parent, sibling or guardian of, or a current or former licensed health care provider of, that woman."[18] Whereas doctors originally were just allowed to challenge laws on the behalf of those who were or could be their patients, this new law allowed a multitude of people to have a say in the process, including physicians who may or may not represent the interests of the person seeking an abortion. In essence, laws that were designed to protect pregnant people at every age, regardless of their inherent chauvinism, were now being used to massively expand the number of interested parties who could make a claim on behalf of the that patient's "best interests," even if it was contrary to the patient's own wishes. Meanwhile, when it came to challenging these laws, those patients couldn't even sue on their own behalf.

•

For Jennie Linn McCormack, what was supposed to be a private, personal decision to do what was best for her family instead turned into a very public nightmare. Word traveled quickly through her small town, and the majority of people turned against her. After her arrest, her mug shot ran in the local paper, a community version of the scarlet letter the prosecutor appeared determined to pin on her. McCormick also lost her job working at the local dry cleaners because neighbors claimed they didn't want her touching their dirty laundry. She was ostracized, and reached a point where she barely left her home. "My neighbors gave me nasty looks when I'd go out in public. They'd get all whispery: 'That's her,'" McCormack told the *Los Angeles Times*. "My kids, they have friends that say stuff to them, and my older two, I feel that they're a little bit ashamed. And that's hard."[19]

While McCormack may not have had much support in her small town, the situation was different nationally, where abortion rights groups filed friend of the court briefs in her favor. Among these groups were the Center for Reproductive Rights, a reproductive rights legal organization that is often involved in challenging state abortion restrictions, and the National Advocates for Pregnant Women, the same group that helped represented Indiana's Bei Bei Shuai in her "feticide" case. Also filing on McCormack's behalf was Legal Voice, a legal advocacy group that argues that if the viability standard presented by *Roe v. Wade* isn't upheld, access to abortion will disappear.

•

The crux of the argument in the Idaho "unlawful abortion" law debate is who should be allowed to perform an abortion—doctors, any medical professional, or the patient themselves? It's a question that, depending on how it is resolved, could literally change the face of abortion access for the entire country. In some ways, the McCormick suit can be seen as the antithesis of medication abortion laws. For example, as we saw in Wisconsin, an attempt to regulate who was allowed to provide RU-486, as well as the protocol that needed to be used to properly administer the medication took a method meant to expand abortion access in rural areas and instead eliminated it by making the law so confusing that no one knew how to legally provide care within the new framework. In McCormack's case, medication abortion was taken to the other extreme: a drug which was completely safe for a patient to use on their own was instead obtained and used with no oversight or follow up. In essence, McCormick herself became the "provider," and abortion opponents made it clear that they were ready to declare her an "illegal" one.

By obtaining medication and undertaking her own abortion, McCormack showed that the medical concerns expressed by abortion opponents who claimed that drugs like RU-486 were dangerous and could not be handled without direct physical supervision was merely a ploy to hamper the abilities of the provider. On the other hand, the case demonstrated why a person also benefitted from medical guidance when terminating a pregnancy. Visiting a clinic would have allowed McCormack to know she was far beyond the gestational cut off for an optimal experience with RU-486. In fact, even at her assumed fourteen weeks gestation, she would not have been approved for the drug. Instead, the clinic would have counseled her on her options at that point, which were either a non-medication abortion or continuing the pregnancy.

However, a clinic abortion of any type wasn't accessible for someone like McCormack. Even if she had had a clinic near her home that should could have used, the financial barriers were too great. The truth was that inducing her own pregnancy at home was always going to be the only option McCormack had if she didn't want to remain pregnant, and that even so late in her pregnancy she had no medical issues with the process—her only real problems were legal.

A person who cannot legally access an abortion isn't likely to simply have a baby, as the McCormack case shows. Quite the opposite; she is likely to go out of her way to terminate the pregnancy—legal, safe or otherwise. Even if the termination is managed without incident, it is apparent from the McCormick case that laws like "illegal abortion" can then be applied at whim to charge pregnant people who are suspected of self-inducing their own miscarriage. And of course when police and prosecutors use their discretion in investigating potential crimes, it is always marginalized communities – especially people of color – who are targeted.

•

In September 2012, the Ninth Circuit Court of Appeals forcefully and unequivocally held that prosecuting McCormack for failing to abide by the state's abortion statutes by obtaining an "unlawful abortion" by buying medications online to terminate her pregnancy was a step too far, in part because it required patients to "police their providers" to assure they were complying with the laws themselves.[20] Judge Harry Pregerson, writing for the majority noted, "Under this Idaho statute, a pregnant woman in McCormack's position has three options: (1) carefully read the Idaho abortion statutes to ensure that she and her provider are in compliance with the Idaho laws to avoid felony prosecution; (2) violate the law either knowingly or unknowingly in an attempt to obtain an abortion; or (3) refrain altogether from exercising her right to choose an abortion."[21]

The decision was remarkable because, for nearly the first time since the Hyde Act, the court took great pains to acknowledge the barriers that pregnant people—especially those who are poor—faced in obtaining abortion services, including lack of providers, financial obstacles, and harassment at clinics. "This Idaho statute heaps yet another substantial obstacle in the already overburdened path that McCormack and pregnant women like her face when deciding whether to obtain an abortion" the court held. Because of the importance of her case, *Newsweek's* Nancy Hass referred to McCormack as "The Next Roe." In the end, though, McCormick never wanted to become a poster child for the abortion movement. She just wanted to make the decision that was best for her family. "My mind just kept going back to my kids, how there was no way I could do that to them, no way I could make their lives even worse."[22]

•

While McCormack was harmed financially and emotionally by her "illegal abortion" experience, she was lucky in comparison to those who came after her. In 2011, anti-abortion forces were just beginning to test out a variety of charges that could be used to prosecute those who terminated pregnancies outside of clinic settings, using homicide, feticide and attempted murder interchangeably.

The most aggressive public and aggressive prosecution occurred in Indiana, where in 2013, Purvi Patel was charged simultaneously with both feticide (causing the death of a fetus in utero) and "neglect of a dependent." Patel was arrested after she went to a hospital emergency room due to excessive bleeding. Upon questioning by an aggressive doctor, who demanded to know if she had just given birth and where the infant was, Patel admitted that she had had a miscarriage, but that the fetus was stillborn so she wrapped it up and placed it in a dumpster. The doctor then left the hospital to personally search for the remains.

After successfully retrieving the body, medical examiners determined that the fetus had taken at least one breath, and therefore must have been alive it was delivered—a claim based on a controversial "lung float" test that many doctors consider inconclusive. Patel was then convicted of both feticide and child neglect, despite the contradiction of the two charges, and sentenced to twenty years in prison. The evidence against her? Texts talking about looking for abortion pills, her "flat demeanor" at the hospital, and her lack of apparent mothering instincts.[23] Patel eventually had both charges overturned in favor of a lesser child neglect conviction, but only after having already spent eighteen months in jail.

Patel wasn't the only person to be turned in by emergency room personnel. In 2015, Kenlissa Jones of Georgia was arrested after going to an ER. after taking medications to end a pregnancy. She was originally charged with "malice murder" before the charges were dropped in exchange for "possession of a dangerous drug."[24] Jennifer Whalen of Pennsylvania was charged with child abuse for obtaining drugs off the internet for her teenage daughter to use when they couldn't find an abortion clinic nearby. Like the others, Whalen was caught when she took her teen in for follow up care at a hospital due to a potential complication. And in what may be the most alarming case, Anna Yocca of Tennessee was arrested and charged with attempted murder when she went to a hospital in fear of her life after attempting to induce her own abortion in a bathtub with a coat hanger. She believed she might be bleeding to death. Instead, the hospital delivered an extremely premature baby and sent Yocca to jail. She eventually pled down to a felony for attempting to terminate her own pregnancy and was released after a year in prison.[25]

Those in the anti-abortion movement have long claimed they have no interest in jailing "mothers" who obtain illegal abortions, and that their only goal is to stop the "illegal abortionists." But as President Donald Trump made clear in his 2016 election campaign, when he said there must be "some punishment" for a person who has an illegal abortion, once pregnant people are their own providers, there is no logical way to separate the two. And as we have seen, in states where abortion is illegal, anti-abortion factions will charge those who terminate their own pregnancies—and those they suspect of doing so, too.

5

INDIANA

CRIMINALIZED PREGNANCIES? WHEN ONE WOMAN'S SUICIDE ATTEMPT BECOMES MURDER

Bei Bei Shuai never believed she would find herself on her knees, sobbing and begging her lover not to leave her. A recent Chinese immigrant, Shuai was nearly eight months pregnant when her boyfriend Zhiliang Guan informed her that he wasn't planning to get a divorce and marry her as he had promised, but was instead returning to his wife. Shuai was heartbroken and believed there was nothing left for her. On December 23, 2010, she left a suicide note saying that she would "take this baby with me to Hades" and ingested rat poison, intending to end her own life.

Luckily, friends discovered Shuai and got her to a hospital, where doctors worked quickly to save her life. While Shuai was physically unharmed, sadly, the same could not be said for her baby. The infant girl Shuai would call "Angel" was monitored in utero for over a week, but on December 31, doctors became concerned for her condition and performed a Caesarean section. Angel came into the world on New Year's Eve at thirty-three weeks gestation. Two days later, she was discovered to have a massive bleed in her brain and was removed from life support.

If Shuai had been brokenhearted after her lover had left her, it was nothing compared to how she felt after the death of her child. After Angel was removed from life support, Shuai held the baby in her arms for the five hours the tiny infant held on, offering in prayer to give up her own life if her daughter could be spared, and demanding that the baby not be taken from her.[1] When Angel died on January 3, 2011, Shuai was immediately transferred to the mental health wing of the hospital, grief-stricken and under heavy sedation. She remained there until March, undergoing treatment. Upon her release, she was charged with murder and thrown in jail.

When Angel died, the coroner indicated the cause of death as the rat poison taken by Shuai, despite the fact that cerebral bleeding is a common condition in many babies born before thirty-four weeks gestation.[2] In addition, Child Protection Services had immediately been alerted when Shuai entered the hospital. Based on these actions, the Indianapolis police arrived at the hospital shortly after Angel's death to conduct interviews to determine whether they would charge Shuai with murder or feticide.[3] In 2009, in response to a robbery that caused a pregnant woman to lose the twins she was carrying, the Indiana House had voted unanimously to strengthen the state's "feticide" law to include any action that caused an unborn child to die, excluding abortion.[4] The law was meant to add additional punishment to crimes that involved pregnant women, with a sentence of up to twenty years in prison if a pregnancy ended as the result of an illegal act. No one had considered that the law could also be used on a pregnant woman herself, especially not one who had committed her own "crime" as a result of mental illness or distress.

At first, the police believed that Shuai had taken the poison not in an attempt to kill herself, but only to terminate her pregnancy. Initial news reports made no mention of suicide, or of her sudden breakup with Guan. The policed didn't even seem sure about a motive behind the act. "It is a very unfortunate situation, very rare circumstances that someone would take rat poison in an attempt to either harm themselves or their unborn baby," said Kendale Adams, public information officer for the Indianapolis Police Department, when discussing the case on the local ABC affiliate a few hours after the investigation had begun.[5] "The fact that there was no licensed physician supervising in a particular case means that the act of abortion is a criminal offense," former Marion County Judge Gary Miller told ABC.[6]

What was most puzzling, however, was why once it became clear that Shuai was indeed trying to end her own life and that terminating a pregnancy wasn't her intention, prosecutors still refused to drop the charges. In fact, the longer the investigation went on, and the more people came to Shuai's defense, the more the state appeared to dig in its heels. Prosecutors claimed they'd thought long and hard about the circumstances before deciding to charge the mourning mother. "This is a very unique case," Dave Rimstidt, Marion County chief trial deputy, told WRTV Indianapolis. "Every charging decision is very difficult and goes through a process where we consider all the facts, all the circumstances, and under this situation, we believe we've charged the two charges we can prove."[7]

In April 2011, Shuai's lawyer, Linda Pence, asked a judge to set bond, a request that was denied. The judge said that no one in the state who had been charged with murder had ever been offered bond in the past, and Shuai's case shouldn't be any different. Pence appealed the ruling in June, but bail was again denied. The judge also denied a motion to dismiss the case, despite a friend of the court brief filed by over eighty pregnancy, women's and civil right groups—including the American College of Obstetricians and Gynecologists—in support of Shuai. "This was a depressed, seriously depressed woman who acted out of an irrational despair and tried to kill herself and, unfortunately, the fetus was harmed,"

Dr. David Orentlicher, a law professor at the Indiana University School of Law and an adjunct professor of medicine at Indiana University School of Medicine, told the local ABC news affiliate. "She had no intent to harm her fetus. That was not the reason she did this."[8]

The basic argument of the prosecution was that the murder and feticide charges were appropriate because the same laws were being applied to Shuai as a pregnant woman as they would be to anyone else who had caused the death of a fetus past viability. Shuai's attorneys and supporters, on the other hand, countered with the claim that the law was being applied to her differently as a pregnant woman, as her actions couldn't be separated from the events that may or may not have caused the death of her baby. Was Shuai in fact being held to a different standard simply by virtue of being pregnant? After all, if she had not been pregnant, and had tried to commit suicide and been saved, the state would not have charged her with attempted murder for trying to kill herself, as suicide itself is not a crime in Indiana. Meanwhile, if the fetus had died in-utero, rather than after it was delivered, Shuai at the very least would not have been looking at a murder charge, and probably would have been granted bail while she awaited trial. And even more ironically, if Shuai had sought an abortion itself eight months into pregnancy and actually found a person willing to provide it, that doctor would have been charged with a crime for committing an illegal abortion, but Shuai herself probably wouldn't have been. Yet here prosecutors were using the suicide as the "crime" on which they were pinning the feticide charge. However, it was because she did everything in her power to save both herself and Angel that Shuai was facing so much time in prison. Emma Ketteringham, then the director of legal advocacy for the National Advocates for Pregnant Women, said that Shuai had been a model patient and mother. "[Shuai] consented to everything the hospital suggested. She agreed to have a C-section and to let the hospital do whatever tests they wanted to do."[9]

In refusing to dismiss the charges against Shuai, the state of Indiana was in essence saying that unborn children had rights, and that those rights outweighed those of the mother carrying it. "Prosecuting women based on the outcomes of their pregnancies violates their constitutional rights and is cruel and unusual punishment. And yet, this is what is happening," wrote author Soraya Chemaly, who followed the Shuai case closely. "In this environment, and with no confidence that their rights will be respected and protected, pregnant women will continue to be jailed, in ever increasing numbers, in unexpected ways that violate their rights. Fear of imprisonment will result in women compromising their health and the health of their fetuses by avoiding pre-natal care, treatment for addiction and medical help if they fear they are miscarrying. They will have more abortions to avoid penalization."[10]

That was why Shuai had no choice but to fight the charges. Constitutional guarantees of due process ensure that no one "may be required at peril of life, liberty or property to speculate as to the meaning of penal statutes. All are entitled to be informed as to what the State commands or forbids." Yet Shuai was denied notice of what the law forbade, as she couldn't have known that attempting suicide would subject her to criminal liability because not even the Indiana legislature had contemplated such an outcome when writing and passing the state's "feticide" law. As her attorneys noted, there was not one single case in Indiana in which a woman had been charged with murder or feticide based solely on allegations that she did or did not do something during pregnancy.[11] Nor had the homicide laws of the state ever been applied to the substantial number of pregnant women who experienced a stillbirth or miscarriage each year, or to other pregnant women in Indiana who had attempted suicide.

Shuai's lawyer Linda Pence accused Marion County Prosecutor Terry Curry of attempting to enforce his own version of the feticide law in order to criminalize the failure to protect a fetus while pregnant. Looking specifically at Shuai's situation, it seems clear that prosecutors were seeking out a "test case" for such a charge. Alerting Child Protective Services when Shuai arrived at the hospital, despite the fact that no child had been born yet, was in itself unusual. That police arrived soon after Angel's death and began interviewing hospital staff was another clue. Curry was accused of building his case solely on an inaccurate, unscientific and discredited autopsy report by a pathologist employed by a private entity named "Biblical Dogs." According to a briefing filed by Shuai's attorneys, the pathologist who performed the autopsy

> offered only a simple inferential analysis of the cause of the baby's hemorrhage based upon nothing more than temporal events and non-medical hearsay statements. In other words, merely because Ms. Shuai ingested poison, that must have caused and thus was the cause of the death of her child. Significantly, the pathologist was not aware that Ms. Shuai had received indomethacin prior to caesarean surgery which has direct side effects upon the fetus alone, including hemorrhaging, and never reviewed Ms. Shuai's medical records, thus precluding her from identifying other issues that could have caused fetal demise, such as a lack of oxygen to the brain. The prosecutor's chief witness did not rule out, nor did she even consider other possible causes of death, never performed research or scientific studies relating to newborn brain bleeds, the effects of blood thinners on persons, pregnant women, or fetuses, nor did she review the medical research in these fields.[12]

Ultimately, Shuai's case left pregnant people exposed to the subjective, scientifically unsound opinions of law enforcement and the state. It also raised severe equal protection concerns as well, since prosecutors effectively made suicide a crime that applied only to pregnant women. Furthermore, a state engages in purposeful gender discrimination when it places additional restrictions on women from which men are exempt, which is unconstitutional under both state and federal law. Shuai did not become pregnant by herself, and in fact, the father of her child, who promised to care for her and their baby and instead abandoned them, was the catalyst of her emotional breakdown. Yet he was not prosecuted despite the fact that "A person who intentionally causes another human being, by force, duress, or deception, to commit suicide commits causing suicide" is a Class B felony in the state of Indiana.[13] The inescapable conclusion of the Shuai case was that in Indiana, a pregnant person now had a fundamentally different relationship to the criminal justice system than did the father of the child.

The right to pro-creational privacy includes the right to carry a pregnancy to term. Indeed, this is the fundamental truth to women's liberty interests: the ability to be free from state-determined procreation. What the state of Indiana was saying with the Shuai prosecution was that people with histories of mental health issues, addictions and other health conditions that might prevent them from being able to ensure a healthy birth outcome, as well as those who could not afford comprehensive prenatal care, drug treatment, and mental health services, could now face prison time if they experienced a miscarriage, stillbirth, or neonatal death. And what happens to those people the state determines are a risk for endangering future pregnancies? In the past, we have forcibly sterilized entire generations of marginalized communities, especially people of color or those with intellectual disabilities. How can we be sure we wouldn't go to a similarly dark place again?

In the end, the most frightening development to come out of the Shaui case was that a judge or jury would be allowed to decide what Shaui's true motive was in trying to end her life—as well as the true motives of anyone in similar circumstance in the future—and put her in jail for up to forty-five years if they sided with the prosecution. The Shuai prosecution represented the logical conclusion of former Justice Kennedy's insistence that the state's primary duty was to protect the rights of potential but unborn life over the rights of person carrying it.

•

Bei Bei Shuai was far from the only woman to fall victim to an overzealous state intent on punishing her for endangering her pregnancy. In March 2010, Iowa mother Christine Taylor fell down a flight of stairs in her home. Taylor, who was pregnant at the time, went to the emergency room to make sure her fetus was okay. While she was in the ER, she spoke with a nurse about her family, including her tumultuous relationship with her husband, the children she already had at home, and the new one on the way. "I never said I didn't want my baby, but I admitted that I had been considering adoption or abortion," Taylor told the *Des Moines Register*. "I admit that I said I wasn't sure I wanted to continue the pregnancy. My husband sends me money, but money doesn't make a parent. I don't have anybody else to turn to."[14] The nurse told a doctor about the conversation, and the doctor in turn called the police, who charged Taylor with "attempted feticide." The charges were later dropped, but only because the feticide law in Iowa applies only to the third trimester, and Taylor was still in her second.

Taylor was lucky. Not so lucky was Rennie Gibbs. In 2006, the sixteen-year-old African-American girl gave birth to a stillborn child at thirty-six weeks. Soon after, it was discovered that Gibbs had used cocaine during her pregnancy. Although there was no proof to tie her drug use to her baby being born dead, Mississippi prosecutors charged the teen as an adult, and accused her of "depraved heart murder" of her child, which has a manda-tory sentence of life in prison. A friend of the court briefing filed on behalf of Gibbs by Tamar Todd of the Drug Policy Alliance and Poonam Juneja of Mississippi Youth Justice Project asked for the dismissal of the charges in May 2010, claiming the "expanded version of the state's homicide statute violates fundamental tenets of common sense and public policy":

> the policy of prosecuting pregnant women and girls with drug dependency or other health problems is contrary to law, scien-tific research, and the consensus judgment of medical practi-tioners and their professional organizations. Furthermore, given the paucity of treatment available in Mississippi, low income women and children would be particularly vulnerable to punish-ment if unable to access drug treatment or prenatal care due to barriers of poverty . . . This prosecution jeopardizes the well-be-ing of women and their children. Interpreting Mississippi's depraved heart murder statute to apply to the context of preg-nancy will lead to absurd and dangerous public health conse-quences. Such prosecutions deter pregnant women from seeking prenatal care and drug and alcohol treatment. And they create a disincentive for pregnant women who do seek medical care from disclosing important information about drug use to health care providers out of fear that the disclosure will lead to possible criminal sanctions. Prosecuting women and girls for continuing to term despite a drug addiction encourages them to terminate wanted pregnancies to avoid criminal penalties.[15]

Gibbs wasn't the first woman to be charged in such a way. National Advocates for Pregnant Women defended over forty women in Texas who were arrested and jailed after a District Attorney decided that under the state's 2003 Prenatal Protection Act, these women could be charged with delivering drugs to "minors" because they abused drugs while pregnant. "While the prenatal protection act was supposed to protect pregnant women, the DA insisted her reading of the statute was justified. Although we were eventually able to overturn the convictions, women spent years in jail while the cases worked their way through the court system," said Lynn Paltrow, NAPW Executive Director.[16]

Texas wasn't the only state to turn pregnant people who used drugs into the human equivalent of meth labs, either. In 2008, Alabama mother Amanda Kimbrough was charged with "chemical endangerment of a child" because she "did knowingly, recklessly, or intentionally cause or permit a child, Timmy Wayne Kimbrough, to be exposed to, to ingest or inhale, or to have contact with a controlled substance, to wit: methamphetamine," according to court records.[17] That "child"? A twenty-one week fetus that was born stillborn after a prolapsed umbilical cord during an extremely premature delivery. Kimbrough's case rose all the way up to the Alabama Supreme Court where, alarmingly, the state decided that not only could the definition of "child" in a child endangerment law refer to the unborn, it could refer to fetus or embryo after the point of conception—a major deviation from precedent when courts usually at least considered viability the standard.

In fact, chemical endangerment laws became a new stopping ground for one segment of the anti-abortion right, with Tennessee adding chemical endangerment to their "fetal assault" law in 2014—a change that explicitly made it a crime to give birth to a child that showed signs of exposure to drugs in utero. The law was withdrawn in 2016 through the co-operative efforts of progressive activists and anti-abortion activists, with abortion opponents concerned that the threat of jail could lead more pregnant people to consider abortion rather than give birth.[18]

•

There's little doubt at this point that a slow but growing faction of society has taken what started out as an interest in protecting a pregnant person and their child and turned that belief on its head by making that person into a potential criminal. From Jennie Linn McCormack's "unlawful abortion" charges and Purvi Patel, Kenlissa Jones and Anna Yocca's "murder" attempts, to the cases of Bei Bei Shuai, Christine Taylor, Rennie Gibbs, and Amanda Kimborough, prosecutors are becoming more willing and comfortable with prosecuting pregnant people for the crime of failing to produce a live pregnancy.[19] Charging women who "didn't protect the fetus," as the prosecutor in McCormack's case called it, is a methodical approach to testing public opinion to see how open the country will be to the idea of criminalizing those who seek illegal abortions once *Roe* is overturned. It also tests the public's appetite when it comes to the potential injuries and even deaths that will occur when pregnant people refuse medical care out of fear of being jailed for a pregnancy that goes wrong—intentionally or not.

This is happening even as anti-abortionists emphasize the framing that "pro-life equals pro-woman" and advance the idea that there are "two victims in every abortion—the mother and the child." Of course, it's not surprising that the increased testing of the water on how palatable the public finds characterizing the "mother" as a "villain" who should be punished for what she has supposedly done to her child is coming hand in hand with a landscape where abortion is less accessible and more people are turning to self-induced terminations outside a legal clinic setting (and without any actual abortion "provider").

It's also no surprise that the majority of those monitored and charged are immigrants, people of color, the poor and other marginalized communities—i.e. those with less resources to defend themselves. These people are also dealing concurrently with racial bias in the medical and legal system, and, thanks to systematic racism, have less available resources for medical care to support a healthy pregnancy to begin with. "Overall as a society, we love to beat up on poor people," explained Pamela Merritt, a reproductive justice activist who often works with communities of color. "Regardless of the fact that we have individual lives and that we are all unique people with experiences, we are a very convenient target. What I see the anti-choice movement doing is they like to co-opt the language. We are only tolerated as victims and so when we're making our reproductive healthcare choices the only way that the abortion is tolerated for black women is if we are some poor, down-trotted victim who doesn't know any better."[20]

The trend is clear, and alarming: under the pretense of "protecting life" more and more states are finding pregnant people criminally liable for pregnancies gone wrong. Much like the push for fetal personhood, feticide prosecutions targeting those who are pregnant effectively strip women of full-legal status and instead place their rights and interests subordinate to those of the fetus. The effect isn't to directly challenge or overturn the right to privacy conferred in *Roe* v. *Wade*—it's to nullify it. "Efforts to re-criminalize abortion and the effort to establish personhood for fertilized eggs, embryos, and fetuses threaten much more than women's reproductive rights," says Lynn Paltrow. "These efforts, if successful will ensure a second class status for all pregnant women and deprive them of their status as persons in the constitutional community....It is important to understand that the attack on 'abortion' and efforts to establish separate legal status for eggs, embryos, and fetuses do not just implicate reproductive rights—but virtually every right, including the right privacy in medical information."

•

After an enormous outpouring of support, as well as pressure on the state, Bei Bei Shuai was finally released on $50,000 bail on May 22, 2012, 435 days after she had been arrested. She moved in with friends and wore an ankle monitor, awaiting her trial date. In July, the prosecution suddenly offered Shuai a deal—plead guilty to feticide, and they wouldn't try her for murder. The offer was tempting. With a feticide plea, though Shuai could conceivably serve twenty years in prison, it could be as little as six, and, if she was highly cooperative, she could receive a suspended sentence. If she didn't take the plea, she could potentially spend most of the rest of her life in prison, if found guilty of murder. Was the prosecution offering a nearly irresistible plea deal in the hope that despite everything, they could still get a feticide precedent on the books? Had the murder charge always been just a threat to get Shuai, a grief-stricken and still new to the country immigrant, to agree to a lesser charge? Whatever the prosecution's motives, Shuai refused the deal. A plea agreement was finally reached in August of 2013. Shuai pled guilty to "criminal recklessness" which was a misdemeanor, and all murder and feticide charges were dropped. [21]

Today, Shuai is free, and the subject of a new documentary about her time fighting felony charges and the injustices people of color and especially immigrant communities face in the legal system. None of this will bring back her baby Angel, but perhaps it can help someone else avoid the agony she has faced.

6

OKLAHOMA

THE SOONER PROBE

To the reproductive rights advocates of Oklahoma, their attempts to fight back against a mandatory ultrasound law must have felt like a Hollywood horror movie: No matter how many times they thought they had slain the monster, it kept popping back up, ready to do battle to the death yet again.

The ultrasound requirement first appeared as part of a 2008 omnibus anti-abortion bill that included, among other anti-abortion legislation, a script for doctors to read to their patients that explained embryonic development; a requirement that doctors make their patients listen to the fetal heartbeat, if possible; a law that protected doctors from so-called "wrongful birth" suits if they refused to tell a patient about potential issues with the fetus to keep them from aborting; and a requirement forcing clinics to post signs regarding the dangers of abortion. Then Governor Brad Henry vetoed the bill, but the state legislature overrode his veto. The courts then blocked the bill prior to enforcement and struck it down all together in August 2009, saying it "violated constitutional requirements that legislative measures deal only with one subject."[1]

That's when the legislature decided to hack the monster into pieces so that it could rise again, reintroducing the omnibus bill as separate bills in 2010. As with the omnibus bill, the smaller bills were vetoed by Henry, whose vetoes were again overridden by the legislature. "Year after year the legislature has passed these really restrictive laws and then the Oklahoma Supreme Court says 'You are violating the state constitution, knock it off,'" remarked Michelle Movahed of the Center for Reproductive Rights, which sued to block the state's ultrasound law. "What they do is they go back into session and they pass the same thing. The sheer disregard for constitutional law and rulings out of the highest arbiter of a state constitutional law is a great example of what's going on here. It's really about chipping away at the various ways in which abortion care can happen in an effort to make it impossible for women to obtain it."[2]

As had been the case with the original set of bills in 2008, it was the mandatory ultrasound bill that received the most attention. The push for mandatory ultrasounds prior to an abortion had started in South Carolina in 2007, though the only requirements were that the procedure be performed (almost always vaginally, since in the first trimester that would provide the more detailed information), and that the patient be offered a chance to look at the results. After becoming law in South Carolina, a dozen states passed similar bills, all using the same "given the opportunity to view the ultrasound" requirement in their respective legislation.[3] States passing the bill implied it was another version of informed consent: A pregnant person can't be fully aware of what pregnancy is, that abortion ends it, and that there really is a life involved unless that person can see it for themselves, they argued. "Ultrasound gives a mother a window to her womb. It helps to prevent her from making a decision she may regret for the rest of her life and it empowers her with the most accurate information about her pregnancy so that she can make a truly informed 'choice,'" said Mary Spaulding Balch of National Right to Life, whose group helped find sponsors for mandatory ultrasound model legislation.[4]

Dr. Curtis Boyd, a long-time abortion provider from even before the passage of *Roe*, was less impressed by the anti-abortion faction's claim to help save pregnant patients from potential "regret":

> The state says, 'We are going to protect you.' And you look where this goes and you see Justice Kennedy said that he felt the state should be allowed to do these things because the woman might regret her decision. Now, whose decision is she going to be allowed to regret? We all may have regrets about decisions we've made, but because you have some regrets doesn't mean that you've made the right or wrong decision. Somehow this woman shouldn't be allowed to make this decision? What if she regrets Justice Kennedy's decision? So he's saying, 'She's not allowed to regret her own decision but she can regret the decision I'm making for her.' That's what it philosophically gets down to.[5]

It was the state of Oklahoma that decided to take the law a step further and force patients to look at the ultrasound pictures whether they wanted to or not, as well as compelling doctors to read a mandatory script regarding fetal development and requiring patients to listen to the baby's heartbeat. The Oklahoma law allowed no exception for women or girls who had been victims of sexual assault, who were told they could just "avert their eyes."[6]

Forcing pregnant patients to view an ultrasound is a strategy that evolved over time. Earlier versions of "Women's Right to Know" ultrasound laws were meant primarily to increase the costs of an abortion to a patient, as well as limit the number of providers by running up the expense of owning a reproductive health care clinic. A majority of the early bills applied only if an ultrasound was used prior to an abortion, and made the requirement of having the patient view the image optional. Alabama then took the additional step in 2002 of requiring that ultrasounds be performed on all patients, and that even clinics that did abortion referrals needed to have an ultrasound machine on site.[7]

To ensure that women had the "right" to view the ultrasound, clinics that provided abortions—or even just offered referrals for them—had to have an ultrasound machine on-site.[8] Ultrasound machines are expensive, however, and crisis pregnancy centers, which often present themselves as full service reproductive health clinics in order to trick patients into entering them rather than abortion clinics, often have them on hand, too. These CPCs push their own ultrasounds on confused patients, hoping that the sight of the fetus will convince them not to go through with having an abortion, and they spend considerable effort on fundraising to have machines on site. Groups like the Knights of Columbus and Focus on the Family gather funds and donations to cover the tens of thousands of dollars necessary to purchase just one machine, putting together charities like "Option Ultrasound" and "Project Ultrasound" for that very purpose.

For "Option Ultrasound," Focus on the Family offers to cover 80 percent of the expense of a new machine for crisis pregnancy centers in "high abortion" communities.[9] The Christian conservative organization announced in October 2011 that it had given away over "528 grants for ultrasound machines or sonography training . . . in 49 states," resulting in "approximately 100,000 women who've seen their baby's ultrasound hav[ing] chosen life."[10] By 2019, the group alleges that that number had increased to "an estimated 425,000 precious moms and their babies!"[11]

In its "Project Ultrasound" program, the national Knights of Columbus offers to match any funds that a state program can raise to purchase machines.[12] One such ultrasound machine was purchased for

North Side Life Care Center in Minneapolis. Executive Director Robbie Dircks told the *Minnesota Christian Examiner*, "I call the ultrasound 'our secret weapon.' That's because once a woman sees her baby and hears the heartbeat, sees it move, I think that there is some bonding that is starting. So instead of wanting to get rid of this thing, now they know that it's just not a blob of flesh—that there really is a baby there. Once a woman has an ultrasound, over 90 percent of them choose life."[13]

Do "90 percent" of pregnant patients really choose to have babies after they've seen an ultrasound? The statistic is cited repeatedly by a myriad of anti-abortion groups, yet the specific talking point is traceable back to a Family Research Council one-page summary on mandatory ultrasound laws, which referred to "an executive director of an Iowa pregnancy resource center" who said that "90 percent of women who see their baby by ultrasound choose life."[14] The FRC summary also cited a variety of other self-reported statistics, all from crisis pregnancy centers, stating that clients are anywhere from "30 percent more likely" to "60 percent more likely" to continue pregnancies, with one pregnancy center stating that, "Ninety-eight percent of women who have ultrasounds chose to carry to term."

However, those who go to crisis pregnancy centers are a self-selected group of patients to begin with. Most who enter these places willingly know that the centers don't perform abortions, and are generally seeking a means to continue their pregnancies. Those who show up by mistake, assuming they are visiting a full services reproductive health clinic, are likely to leave before they ever get to the ultrasound portion of the appointment. That the vast majority of people who go to pregnancy centers and see ultrasounds choose not to get an abortion shouldn't be surprising at all, but those numbers aren't replicated in patients who go to reproductive health clinics to procure a termination. Although no studies have been done in the United States, a 2010 *New York Times* article stated that clinics in British Columbia reported that no patients changed their minds about terminating a pregnancy after viewing an ultrasound, and anecdotal evidence from providers in the US tell of the same experience.[15]

In the wake of the passage of mandatory ultrasound laws, crisis pregnancy clinics are being trained to do whatever it takes to get pregnant people in the door, even if it means telling them that they will need an ultrasound before an abortion, and that the ones they offer are free.

What they don't mention, however, is that the ultrasound required by law has to be performed by the patient's own provider prior to the termination, and that the one at the pregnancy center doesn't count. In a workshop called "Competing with the Abortion Industry," former Planned Parenthood employee turned anti-abortion spokeswoman Abby Johnson explained to owners and volunteers at pregnancy centers how to best get clients into their clinics. "Who's your demographic? Abortion-minded clients, right?" Johnson said during the training. "We want to look professional, we want to look business-like, and yeah, we do kind of want to look medical. We want to appear neutral on the outside. The best call, the best client you ever get is one who thinks they are walking into an abortion clinic." Johnson went on to describe the best way to get those who mistakenly believe they are walking into an abortion clinic to submit to an ultrasound. "What I would encourage you to do is say something like this. 'No, we do not provide abortion services, but we do provide ultrasounds, and you are going to need an ultrasound before you have your abortion.' And that's true. You want them in your center that day. You want to say, 'Well, no, we don't actually provide abortion procedures here, but we do provide ultrasounds and that's one of the steps of having an abortion so you can come in here and you can get your ultrasound done for free. Because you're going to have to do it anyway when you have an abortion.' The goal is to get them into your center as quickly as possible."[16]

As Johnson's talk shows, for those who oppose abortion, mandatory ultrasounds are an opportunity. For those who hold the pregnant patient's health as the priority, however, mandatory ultrasounds harm those who want to terminate a pregnancy by taking away their feelings of autonomy. Dr. Tracy Weitz, Associate Director for Public Policy at the UCSF National Center of Excellence in Women's Health, wrote that

> By mandating that they view the image and hear a script in accordance with the desires of the state legislature, women's own preferences are ignored. Removing women's ability to decide whether to have an ultrasound before an abortion and dictating the manner in which the ultrasound is administered is likely to reduce women's perceptions of decisional control regarding abortion, and thus may have negative psychological and physical health outcomes, impede adjustment, and increase the risk of decisional regret in all women seeking abortions under such conditions.[17]

Over the governor's objections, Oklahoma's mandatory forced ultrasound bill became law on April 27, 2010. The law was only active for a few days before a temporary restraining order was enacted that allowed clinics to stop complying while the legal challenges occurred, due to an agreement between the state's attorney general and the Center for Reproductive Rights, which was challenging the law as unconstitutional.

In those few days that the law was in effect, however, something became very clear; namely that the "90 percent of women" who "choose life" obviously only went to crisis pregnancy centers. For example, one clinic in Tulsa, which also had an adoption center on-site, reported that not a single patient who saw an ultrasound changed their mind about having an abortion. Executive Director Linda Meeks of Reproductive Services told *NewsOK* that some closed their eyes, turned their heads away, or even cried after seeing the picture, but none chose not to terminate. "It's like [lawmakers] don't think women have given serious thought and consideration before they walk through our doors."[18]

With the restraining order in place, the courts continued to bat around at the mandatory ultrasound law until Judge Bryan Dixon ruled that it should be permanently blocked, calling it unconstitutional, since it applied only to abortion and no other medical procedures. Dixon said the law "improperly is addressed only to patients, physicians and sonographers concerning abortions and does not address all patients, physicians and sonographers concerning other medical care where a general law could clearly be made applicable."[19]

That should have been the end of the bill, but it wasn't. Unable to let the monster rest, Oklahoma Attorney General Scott Pruitt (later head of the Environmental Protection Agency under President Trump, until he resigned under a cloud of scandal in 2018) filed an appeal to the Oklahoma Supreme Court asking that it invalidate the ruling. "Understood in its most basic terms, the trial court—in error—ruled that the Oklahoma Constitution forbids legislation ensuring women receive meaningful medical information obtained through ultrasounds that the clinics are currently requiring," Pruitt wrote.[20]

Why would the state of Oklahoma be so unwilling to let the bill go away? One obvious answer was that abortion opponents needed the federal courts to disagree on the issue, as splitting the circuit courts would prompt the US Supreme Court to step in and settle the dispute.

•

While the Oklahoma challenge worked its way through the state court system, similar bills in Texas and North Carolina lined up to help to grease the wheels. In Texas, forcing pregnant people to undergo and view an ultrasound prior to having an abortion wasn't just a mission, it was supposedly also an emergency. The Texas senate introduced its own mandatory forced ultrasound bill in February 2011, and Republican Governor Rick Perry (who would announce plans to run for the GOP presidential nomination six months later) fast tracked it as an "emergency priority bill." "Considering the magnitude of the decision to have an abortion, it is crucial that Texans understand what is truly at stake," Perry said in a released statement.[21]

Although Perry considered the bill a priority, Judge Sam Sparks of the US District Court for the Western District of Texas considered it a serious violation of the first amendment. After rejecting numerous "friend of the court" briefs from anti-abortion groups and chastising lawyers for wasting his time ("The Court has already turned down two extremely tempting offers to transform this case from a boring old federal lawsuit into an exciting, politically-charged media circus. As any competent attorney could have predicted, the Court declines this latest invitation as well,") Sparks struck down the law.[22] The judge said the bill, "compels physicians to advance an ideological agenda with which they may not agree, regardless of any medical necessity, and irrespective of whether the pregnant women wish to listen," constituting state-sanctioned speech and a clear violation of the first amendment.[23]

Just is in Oklahoma, the state of Texas appealed the ruling. But unlike Oklahoma, the state of Texas received a far different result when a three-judge panel on the Fifth Circuit overturned Sparks' ruling, with then Chief Justice Edith Jones ruling that opponents of the law "failed to demonstrate constitutional flaws" in the bill. The Fifth Circuit Court of Appeals, which hears cases from Texas, Mississippi and Louisiana, is known to be among the most conservative appellate districts in the country, and this is in large part due to Jones, who was Chief Justice until 2012, and is still on the bench. Under her leadership, the Fifth Circuit has taken a very harsh line with regards to women's issues. This is a court that, for example, sanctioned a cheerleader for suing her school district after she was forced to cheer for a student who had sexually assaulted her. Jones is also known for blistering dissents, particularly when it comes to women's rights. One of her dissents stated that a woman needed to be raped to claim actual sexual harassment, while in another she told a molestation victim that there was no legal benefit in recognizing "a constitutional right not to have her bodily integrity compromised by a teacher's sexual abuse."[24] Female bodily autonomy is clearly not a priority for Justice Jones, which made her the prefect appellate judge for the anti-abortion movement's challenge to the ultrasound law.

In her ruling, Jones said that if states could require abortion providers to give patients illustrated pamphlets showing the development of the fetus, as long as the information was "truthful and non-misleading" they could "empower" those same patients with even better, more specific and technologically advanced imaging. Jones held that a sonogram image was the "epitome" of truthful information, even if it is more graphic than the informational pamphlets showing the development of fetuses that *Casey* approved. "Only if one assumes the conclusion of Appellees' argument, that pregnancy is a condition to be terminated, can one assume that such information about the fetus is medically irrelevant." Jones held. "The point of informed consent laws is to allow the patient to evaluate her condition and render her best decision under difficult circumstances. Denying her up to date medical information is more of an abuse to her ability to decide than providing the information."[25]

While Jones considered the ultrasound "empowering" for pregnant patients seeking abortions, the Center for Reproductive Rights disagreed. "The Texas law was addressing a problem that didn't exist because women always had the option to view an ultrasound before obtaining their abortions if they wanted to," said Michelle Mohaved. "What the Texas law did was remove the agency from the women and put it in the hands of the state. So it says 'You are not smart enough to make the choice yourself about whether you should see the ultrasound. We've decided for you.' If it was about empowering women, you would support all sorts of choices."[26]

While Jones and her colleagues may have ruled mandatory forced ultrasounds as "reasonable," and "empowering" to patients, for providers, it was a clear violation of medical best practices. Dr. Curtis Boyd, who provides abortions under the new mandatory ultrasound law, describes the dilemma abortion providers now face in caring for patients. "The state mandated information is part of informing the patient. Well, some of this information is erroneous. Some of it is exaggerated or inaccurate and some of it is just out and out wrong but we're required to give it," he said. "You have the state intervening and mandating to doctors that they give specific information to their patient which the doctor of medicine in general may not agree with and may in fact clearly disagree with. Yet the state says 'If you don't do this, you're subject to losing your medical license.' So I have to do it. Well, you say don't do it but it's unethical. If I don't and I provide the service, I'm subject to having my license revoked and having a felony filed against me. In fact, I am coerced just as a woman is."[27]

•

As the Texas challenge was snaking its way through the Fifth Circuit, another ultrasound law from North Carolina was simultaneously working through the Fourth Circuit Court of Appeals. Under North Carolina's law, a doctor must perform an ultrasound on a pregnant patient seeking an abortion and then display the images, noting "the presence, location, and dimensions of the unborn child" and describing "external members and internal organs, if present and viewable." Several North Carolina doctors and health care providers challenged the constitutionality of the law in the case of *Stuart v. Huff*.

Judge Catherine Eagles of the US District Court for the Middle District of North Carolina preliminarily enjoined the "speech-and-display requirements," of the law, as she called them. "The First Amendment," she wrote, "generally includes the right to refuse to engage in speech compelled by the government." The North Carolina ultrasound law required speech via words and imagery, "even when the provider does not want to deliver the message and even when the patients affirmatively do not wish to see it or hear it," Eagles wrote. She also found "no medical purpose" in the speech-and-display requirements.[28] In December 2014, the Fourth Circuit Court of Appeals upheld that decision, and in June 2015, the Supreme Court declined to step in, leaving the North Carolina decision blocked.

To date, the Supreme Court has refused to step back into the fight over the balance of rights between state restrictions on abortions and a doctor's speech rights in the practice of medicine. In *Bigelow v. Virginia* (1975), the Court ruled that the First Amendment protects abortion advertisements, and that states can't prevent publishers from running ads for abortion services. Jeffrey Bigelow, editor of *The Virginia Weekly*, had published an ad for a New York agency offering to connect women in Virginia (where abortion law was more restrictive) with abortion doctors in New York (where abortion law was more permissive). He was convicted under a Virginia law that made it a crime to "encourage or prompt the procuring of abortion." Bigelow filed suit claiming the law violated his First Amendment right to free speech. The Supreme Court overturned his conviction, noting that the First Amendment gives some protection even to commercial speech, concluding that the abortion ad was entitled to protection because it promoted services that were legal in New York and contained information of "constitutional interest" to the general public.[29]

The Court later took up the specific issue of regulating doctor's speech and First Amendment rights in *Casey*, finding that legislatures can mandate doctors provide "truthful, nonmisleading information about the nature of the procedure, the attendant health risks and those of child-birth, and the 'probable gestational age" of the fetus in a way that prevents compelling speech.[30] But while it dealt with the issue generally, the Court did not address what level of scrutiny courts must employ when analyzing speech claims such as these, therefore leaving open the question of just how specific legislatures can script medical disclosures in the name of restricting access to abortion.

Compelled speech or not, some doctors are still searching for a way to balance the rights of patients to get accurate information with the state's decision to press a script upon them. Dr. Boyd has his own way of reconciling the two—he provides the state script, then adds his own thoughts at the end of it:

> Sometimes I wonder what would happen if the state wanted to make an issue of it, You know, 'We've already told you what you must say, now you can't say . . .' I don't know. They can't rule that I can't have an opinion. They have sort of ruled what my opinion must be to the patient, but it doesn't say clearly you can't tell the patient you think something differently. So I do it. I think 'Well, they'll just have to take me to court.' There's just a limit to how far they can go. I have to salvage my integrity somehow. So I say 'This is what the state wants me to tell you and my own belief is that abortion does not cause breast cancer' and so forth. And that you are quite ethically confident to make this decision.

I respect your decision-making process. I've given you the decision-making process the state wants you to follow.

For abortion opponents trying to either coerce pregnant patients into continuing their pregnancies directly, or provoke a Supreme Court challenge that could overturn *Roe*, the Texas situation couldn't have turned out much better. But for those who have actually had to undergo a mandatory forced ultrasound, it's a different story. Reporter Carolyn Jones wrote about her own brush with the mandatory forced ultrasound bill in Texas, after learning that the baby she had carried for twenty weeks had a terminal anomaly and was unlikely to survive past birth. Although she technically should have been exempt from the verbal description and waiting period portion of the bill, providers were so confused as to what was and wasn't legally necessary at that point that she became subject to it anyway.

In an article in the *Texas Observer*, Jones explained the horror of being forced against her will to listen to a description of the fetus, while her doctor apologized for his part in her suffering. He didn't want to give her this information, but his hands were tied. It was the law.

'I'm so sorry that I have to do this,' the doctor told us, 'but if I don't, I can lose my license.' Before he could even start to describe our baby, I began to sob until I could barely breathe. Somewhere, a nurse cranked up the volume on a radio, allowing the inane pronouncements of a DJ to dull the doctor's voice. Still, despite the noise, I heard him. His unwelcome words echoed off sterile walls while I, trapped on a bed, my feet in stirrups, twisted away from his voice. 'Here I see a well-developed diaphragm and here I see four healthy chambers of the heart . . .' closed my eyes and waited for it to end, as one waits for the car to stop rolling at the end of a terrible accident.[31]

Her ultrasound ended, and like nearly all women forced into mandatory ultrasounds, Jones had her termination.

•

In 2012, an Oklahoma state judge eventually agreed with abortion rights supporters and permanently blocked the state's mandatory ultrasound bill, calling the law an unconstitutional violation of free speech.[32] That left Texas as the only state able to put the ban in effect, and should have stopped copycat bills from being filed—or becoming law.

It didn't work. According to the Guttmacher Institute, as of 2019, twelve states mandated ultrasounds prior to an abortion, although only four of those make the provider also show the ultrasound and describe what is seen in the image. Kentucky was the latest to join that group, as the Sixth Circuit Court of Appeals ruled in April of 2018 that the state's mandatory ultrasound bill—which requires the doctor to narrate the ultrasound and play the heartbeat of the embryo or fetus—was not a violation of the free speech rights of the provider. "The information conveyed by an ultrasound image, its description and the audible beating fetal heart gives a patient a greater knowledge of the unborn life inside her," wrote Judge John Bush, a Trump appointee. "This also inherently provides the patient with more knowledge about the effect of an abortion procedure: it shows her what or whom she is consenting to terminate."[33] Another eleven states simply mandate an ultrasound, although no narration is necessary, and nine of those demand the patient be provided the opportunity to view the ultrasound although it does not require the patient to look at it.[34]

The fact that only four states are forcing patients to listen to a narrated ultrasound may seem like at least a small victory against compulsory government-mandated speech. However, many state legislatures have struck another blow against free speech through a completely different avenue—so-called "informed consent" laws that are tacked onto mandatory waiting periods. And this time they aren't taking no for an answer. Though abortion opponents never quite managed to get the Supreme Court to bite on the split circuit decision that evolved from mandatory ultrasound bills, like the monster of all horror movies, these compelled speech requirements simply found a new landscape from which to rise again. And, like their horror film counterparts, no matter how many times they are struck down, they just keep coming back to life.

7

SOUTH DAKOTA

COME FOR THE ABORTION, STAY FOR
THE CONVERSION TO CHRISTIANITY

Leslee Unruh made it clear that sexual activity of any form outside of the marriage bed was physically and emotionally damaging, a fact that she believed most of the world failed to recognize. As the spokeswoman for Abstinence Clearinghouse, a South Dakota-based organization that "promotes the appreciation for and practice of sexual abstinence through distribution of age-appropriate, factual and medically-accurate materials," her crusade was to spread the gospel of abstinence until marriage, as well as tell the world that pornography, homosexuality (even if monogamous) and masturbation were harmful to the person engaging in these activities.

But if Abstinence Clearinghouse and abstinence-only education was Unruh's crusade, it was her pregnancy center, Alpha Center, that was her kingdom. There, Unruh tended to those who had unexpectedly become pregnant, allowing her access to potential souls to save, babies to bring into the world, and financial profit, too. While Unruh spent the 1990's telling young girls to wear purity rings to protect them from premarital sex, in the 1980s, she had run a maternity home known as the Omega

House, where she cared for unwed mothers. According to a *More* magazine profile on Unruh, it was one year after Omega House opened that Alpha Center was accused of offering potential mothers money to continue their pregnancies and then give their babies up for adoption after they were born. The center was charged with twenty-four counts of unlicensed adoption and foster care practice as well as false advertising, although most of the charges were dismissed after Unruh pled no contest to five counts and paid a $500 fine.[1]

Despite this, Alpha Center lived on, providing support for those who wanted to give birth to their unplanned babies while also trying to coax and in some cases trick pregnant people who believed they had entered an abortion clinic into not terminating their pregnancies. Business was good—the organization received $2 million in taxpayer dollars between 2004 and 2009 for its abstinence only sex education programs.[2] Unruh had successfully turned abstinence into a profitable enterprise. And while she had long been highly involved in lobbying for abortion restrictions in South Dakota, once the state attempted to ban abortion completely, she became even more engrossed in legislative efforts.

Though a total ban on abortion in South Dakota had failed in 2006, anti-abortion activists tried again in 2008, with Unruh spearheading the "Vote Yes for Life" campaign, which would ban almost all abortions (though it allowed narrow exceptions for pregnancies that were a result of rape, incest, or that threatened a pregnant person's life.) When asked why she was pushing a ban two years after the voters had rejected one, Unruh explained, "I don't think they gave their final word."[3] The voters disagreed with her, as the ban was voted down again and abortion opponents were forced to look for a new restriction that would be more palatable to the general public.

To the rescue came state representative Roger Hunt, who in 2011 proposed H.B. 1217, a bill that he said would ensure that the choice to terminate a pregnancy was "voluntary, uncoerced, and informed.[4]" The "coerced abortion" idea was a favorite of Hunt's, a rabid opponent of a abortion rights. For example, Hunt was very vocal in explaining why exceptions for rape, incest and health were left out of the 2006 total abortion ban: women lie. In a 2006 interview with *Time* magazine, Hunt explained his stance: If a woman really was raped, she could go to the hospital and take emergency contraception the night of the attack. In that instance, using emergency contraception (which he seemed to believe caused an abortion) would be justified. But if the state allowed a general exception for rape, how could it know a woman wasn't just claiming to be raped in order to obtain a pregnancy termination?

> So why not have an exemption for all rape victims, including the ones who are too shattered to report an assault right away? Hunt calls it "a fine line that we're walking, but some of this is just to show that we're being fair and reasonable. In cases where we cannot determine if there's an unborn child or not, we're trying to be sympathetic to a woman who alleges she's been raped." But the sympathy expires after about a week. Very honestly, Hunt adds, "We don't want to have a lot of abortion clinics questioning a woman and having the woman say 'well, I was raped four months ago, I need an abortion.' We're trying to be sensitive to women who are legitimate rape victims—and not give abortion clinics a chance to commit fraud on system."[5]

As for coercion, Hunt believed that almost every person considering abortion was being pressured by someone. "She may be dealing with a lot of pressure, from family, boyfriend, husband. We have a situation in which the woman may be getting so much pressure she's not thinking clearly," he told *Time*.[6]

Hunt's proposed bill would have taken the state's mandatory twenty-four-hour waiting period in between the patient meeting with a doctor and having the abortion and stretch it to seventy-two hours. It would also have compelled a face to face meeting with a doctor, which would add an additional physical trip for women to the state's only clinic, located in Sioux Falls. On its own, changing the waiting period from one to three days was a huge issue for a state that had one abortion clinic. According to Alisha Sedor, then the Executive Director of NARAL Pro-Choice South Dakota, the Sioux Falls clinic was convenient for the large number of state residents that lived in the area, but for the rest of South Dakotans, it was often easier to leave the state all together. "While this is the largest metropolis in the state, there are women that live in Rapid City which is five hours away," she said. "If they were interested in accessing abortion services in South Dakota they'd have to drive ten hours round trip and if this law goes into effect they would have to do that potentially three times. So that's quite a bit of road time. There are certainly a number of women who leave the state just because it's easier, less travel, and less hoops to jump through in order to obtain services."[7]

Though forcing pregnant people to leave the state to access abortion was obviously fine with South Dakota legislators like Roger Hunt, it would be a great hardship for the rural poor of the state. "Obviously women who are low income and live in rural areas, they have to travel further and spend more," said Sedor. "If you don't have the resources to do that, then you don't have access to services at all, if you can't access the funds to travel to Sioux Falls or out of state." The most likely group to be impacted by an extended waiting period would be residents of South Dakota's Indian reservations, where health care access was already difficult to obtain. "Anecdotally, I think that women on the reservation, Native women are impacted more so than others because the reservations are located in some of the poorest counties in the country," said Sedor. "Not only do they lack resources, but also information and there's very little access to services on the reservation. That is extremely problematic from our point of view because you're impacting minority and low-income women more than anyone else."

Lakota reproductive rights activist Sunny Clifford was well-aware of the problems the Native American community in the state already had in accessing family planning and reproductive health care. "Women on the Pine Ridge Reservation face great distances between their homes and clinics," said Clifford, a Pine Ridge resident and former board member for NARAL Pro-Choice South Dakota. "Some women are fortunate enough to live near the hospital or clinics, but there are some who must find a way to travel up to sixty miles, one way. Not everybody on the reservation owns a vehicle and if there is vehicular access then they must find the gas money, which isn't always there. We do have a public transit system and a lot of people utilize that, but access is only on weekdays. Also, clinics and access to the women's health clinic is only available on certain days of the week."[8] According to Clifford, adding in a seventy-two-hour waiting period would make accessing abortion become nearly impossible for community members:

> Let's say a woman from the reservation is seeking an abortion. If the woman is from Pine Ridge reservation she has to find a way to get to Sioux Falls, which is a five hour trip. She's already on a time limit. Then when she gets there she must go through mandatory counseling and then wait seventy-two hours and in the meantime provide herself lodging when she probably barely had enough money just to make it to Sioux Falls. The

seventy-two-hour wait places unnecessary struggles on Native American women with little money and little time. What if by trying to get enough money she was then running up against the legal limit to have an abortion? Those additional seventy-two hours could very well make her ineligible.

While the extended wait time and additional travel expenses were a problem, it was the bill's other requirement that really got reproductive rights and civil rights supporters up at arms. Under H.B. 1217, as part of the new standard for pre-abortion care, a pregnant person would be forced to enter a crisis pregnancy center (CPC), and allow the volunteers inside to try and to talk them out of terminating the pregnancy. According to the bill:

> [P]rior to the day of any scheduled abortion the pregnant mother must have a consultation at a pregnancy help center at which the pregnancy help center shall inform her about what education, counseling, and other assistance is available to help the pregnant mother keep and care for her child, and have a private interview to discuss her circumstances that may subject her decision to coercion. That prior to signing a consent to an abortion, the physician shall first obtain from the pregnant mother, a written statement that she obtained a consultation with a pregnancy help center, which sets forth the name and address of the pregnancy help center, the date and time of the consultation, and the name of the counselor at the pregnancy help center with whom she consulted.[9]

If there was any doubt that the intent of the bill was to ensure that a pregnant person was talked out of her decision to have an abortion, it was dispelled by the bill's definition of a "pregnancy center."

The pregnancy help center has a facility or office in the state of South Dakota in which it routinely consults with women for the purpose of helping them keep their relationship with their unborn children; that one of its principal missions is to educate, counsel, and otherwise assist women to help them maintain their relationship with their unborn children; that they do not perform abortions at their facility, and have no affiliation with any organization or physician which performs abortions; that they do not now refer pregnant women for abortions, and have not referred any pregnant women for an abortion at any time in the three years immediately preceding July 1, 2011.[10]

The greatest concern for activists in South Dakota was that under the guise of making sure a patient wasn't being coerced into having an abortion, pregnancy centers would instead be acting to coerce that patient out of one. "Often crisis pregnancy centers are religiously affiliated, they are explicitly anti-choice and their sole goal is to talk women out of seeking services," said Sedor. "In some cases it's abortions and in others it's abortion and birth control and anything else that has to do with healthy sexuality. In this case, I think that this legislation was brought with hope that, if women are forced to walk in the door of these places that they will be able to inundate them with anti-choice rhetoric and talk them out of seeking the services that they are looking to find. It also left these crisis pregnancy centers relatively unregulated in what they can and can't say to women. So there's nothing to say that they just can't out and out lie. Our fear is that, while this legislation talks about women who are coerced into abortions, that their goal is to actually coerce women out of having them even if that's a decision that's right for them and their family."

The bill did make it clear that the pregnancy center "counselors" doing the coercion evaluation wouldn't be conducting religious conversions at the same time by mandating that the counselors could only discuss religion if the client first signed a form in agreement. Still, there was no doubt that under the bill, those seeking terminations would be forced into dealing with faith-based organizations. As Allen Unruh, Leslee Unruh's husband and co-founder of Alpha Center explained, the "entire Alpha Center story was inspired by God, and the rising up of Godly people with courage to be salt and light; to take action against the most evil act in this generation—the killing of innocent unborn babies and the deliberate deception of millions of women."[11]

Planned Parenthood condemned H.B. 1217 as a bill designed to force pregnant patients to discuss basic medical care with a person who had no medical background. "This bill, the first of its kind in the nation, would require women in some of the most difficult circumstances, including victims of rape and incest and mothers facing serious complications, to get permission for a legal medical procedure from an unregulated agency staffed by untrained volunteers," stated Sarah Stoesz, CEO of Planned Parenthood Minnesota, North Dakota, South Dakota. "It's outrageous that the state would mandate that a woman must seek permission from a so-called crisis pregnancy centers, which are not legitimate medical facilities, before she could access safe, legal abortion care from her doctor."[12]

It wasn't just seeking permission, either, as Alisha Sedor explained. Crisis pregnancy centers would also have personal and contact information on every person in the state seeking an abortion. Although an updated version of H.B. 1217 required that they keep the information confidential, it still provided no penalties if the center did not. "There is nothing that can be done if, let's say, that information was released," Sedor said. "It also just says that they can't release the information, it doesn't say what they can't do with it themselves. So they certainly can continue to reach out to these women and you can just imagine a slew of ways in which they harass and shame these women out of receiving services. It's certainly scary, an explicitly anti-choice organization in the middle of a woman and her physician as she's trying to obtain these completely legal services."

The bill angered not just the standard reproductive rights advocates, but civil rights groups as well. Americans United was concerned that the state might in fact be legislating religion on top of violating medical rights to privacy. "There has been some talk about challenging this provision of South Dakota's law in court," wrote Americans United's Rob Boston. "I hope that happens. I also hope it is struck down as a violation of the fundamental right of conscience."[13] The South Dakota chapter of the American Civil Liberties Union vowed to fight the bill in court if it were ever signed into law, joining Planned Parenthood.

If the opposition from these two groups was expected, opposition from another corner was much more surprising, as a large number of pregnancy centers didn't support the bill, either. Some worried that providing a patient with forms verifying that they met would make them complicit in the abortion itself. "[W]e are not here to talk women into or out of anything. We are here to make it possible for women to carry to term if that's what they want to do in their heart of hearts," Bella Pregnancy Center executive director Roxanne Johnson told *The Rapid City Journal*. "Because I have seen firsthand the devastation that abortion has caused many women and families, I would have a difficult time providing any statement that would assist or facilitate an abortion."[14] Leslee Unruh seemed less concerned, saying that the centers weren't complicit since the patient could always lie. "The woman can walk in the door and walk out without talking to anybody and say she was there. It's an honor system."[15]

Unruh may have been ready to move on the bill, but Republican Dennis Daugaard, who served as governor of South Dakota from 2011 to 2019, wasn't quite as anxious, as the state was already defending other abortion restrictions that had been proposed, passed and then blocked by the courts. As a result, the state was incurring hundreds of thousands of dollars in legal fees, and if they lost this fight, they would be responsible for paying the plaintiff's legal bills as well. South Dakota had already paid about $500,000 to Planned Parenthood for legal fees in prior years, and Daugaard didn't want to run up another tab. It took nearly two weeks after the passage of the bill before Daugaard finally signed it into law. The governor gave no interviews, but said in a statement, "I hope that women who are considering an abortion will use this three-day period to make good choices."[16]

The reason for the lag time between the bill's passage and Daugaard's signature was because the governor knew the law would end up in court, and he was thus unwilling to sign it until he knew who was going to pay for the litigation. Once again, Representative Roger Hunt came to the rescue. If Daugaard would sign the bill, Hunt promised he would solicit donations to a legal fund the state could then use to pay for the expected litigation. "They want to put their money where their mouth is in the sense of protecting unborn children," Hunt said of the donations his group received.[17] Lawmakers, even Republican ones, were less excited by the prospect of anonymous or outside forces paying for the state's legal expenditures. "Either the state of South Dakota believes as a matter of policy that this is what we do and we pay for it or we don't," said Senator Joni Culter, a Republican from Minnehaha County. "When we open the door for outsiders to come in and pay for it, that's just bad. When we're using the state's resources to litigate private matters just because someone claims someone else is going to drop a coin into a bucket, that's just bad government."[18]

Ultimately, some money flowed into the fund, but not a great amount. During the week surrounding Daugaard's signing of the bill on

March 28, 2011 and Hunt's pledge to solicit donors, the fund gained about $15,000. Most of the money came from small pledges, though a few bigger donations came from people that were actively involved with Leslee Unruh's "Vote Yes" campaign, such as Dr. Patricia Giebink and Todd and Linda Broin. A donation of $2,500 came from the Gerard Health Foundation, best known for funding the Lila Rose and Live Action and their inaccurate attack videos attempting to discredit, defund and otherwise shut down Planned Parenthood.[19] Most interesting were two small donations. One, a twenty-dollar anonymous donation, was a reminder that unlike campaign donations, there was no requirement to disclose where the money came from. Another $100 came from Allen Unruh, Leslee's husband and co-founder of Alpha Center.[20]

•

Planned Parenthood of Minnesota, North Dakota, South Dakota and the ACLU both followed through on their promise to challenge H.B. 1217. There are two ways to challenge abortion laws like these: on their face, or as they are applied. Facial challenges usually carry a more difficult burden because plaintiffs have to show that in a "large fraction" of the cases in which the relevant law would be applied, a substantial obstacle to a pregnant person's decision to undergo an abortion would be present. However, to challenge as applied would mean waiting until after the law had gone into effect.

Not wanting pregnant people to be forced to violate either their privacy or their civil rights in order to terminate a pregnancy, Planned Parenthood and the ACLU had no choice but to challenge the suit on its face. The two groups filed suit on May 27, 2011, blocking the bill well before its scheduled start date of July 1. "The Act has both the purpose and the effect of severely restricting access to health care, and violates patients' and physicians' First Amendment rights against compelled speech and patients' right to privacy in their personal and medical information," said Planned Parenthood Federation of America attorney Mimi Liu when announcing the suit.[21]

For his part, Roger Hunt confessed to not comprehending what all the fuss was about. "I don't understand why [they are suing], because it just seeks to give women more information and it seeks to remove coercion, seeks to deal with a number of coercion elements where you have possible rapes and problems within families and what not, and we're trying to help those women deal with that coercion," he told the Associated Press. "All of that seems to me to be in support of women, but for some reason Planned Parenthood sees their money supply and the abortions being dried up so obviously they're going to fight."[22]

Hunt may not have understood why the groups were suing, but US District Court Chief Judge Karen Schreier certainly did. She ruled that the law would remain blocked, and that compelling pregnant people to visit pregnancy health centers was likely unconstitutional. "Forcing a woman to divulge to a stranger at a pregnancy help center the fact that she has chosen to undergo an abortion humiliates and degrades her as a human being. The woman will feel degraded by the compulsive nature of the Pregnancy Help Center requirements, which suggest that she has made the 'wrong' decision, has not really 'thought' about her decision to undergo an abortion, or is 'not intelligent enough' to make the decision with the advice of a physician. Furthermore, these women are forced into a hostile environment."[23]

Following Schreier's ruling, Alpha Center and another South Dakota pregnancy center successfully sued to intervene in the case. Their reasoning was that, "[b]ecause there are about 700 abortions performed in South Dakota annually . . . they could be denied access to that many clients by

Planned Parenthood's lawsuit."[24] Much as Jennie Linn McCormack's lawyer Rick Hearn had intervened on her behalf in Idaho as a physician who
could potentially provide care and be affected by the abortion ban he was
challenging, the crisis pregnancy centers had decided to step in as a new
type of "provider" who could intervene on behalf of pregnant people as
potential patients. Once more, the definition of a provider and medical
entity was being turned on its head.

The challenge to H.B. 1217 raised a series of important issues in
the clash between reproductive rights and the practice of medicine. At
the heart of the case was the issue of informed consent. According to
Planned Parenthood v. Casey, because an informed consent requirement
must "facilitate the wise exercise" of a pregnant person's right to abortion,
such a requirement presents an undue burden unless it provides "truthful and not misleading" information.[25] The legal principle seems simple and straightforward: if government is going to mandate that doctors
disclose certain information to patients in the course of rendering medical treatment, that information must be truthful. But since *Gonzales v.
Carhart* declared that legislatures could craft law in areas where there was
no medical consensus, what does it mean to have a "truthful" disclosure?
The question would presumably coalesce with medical standards of care
in treating pregnant people. But that hasn't been the case, in large part
because of the impact of the *Gonzales* decision and a shift in the court to
deferring to legislators over doctors when dictating what information a
patient needs to know prior to making a decision to abort.

The legal battles over the contours of "informed consent" and "truth"
as determined by anti-abortion rights legislatures dates back to 2005
and initial legal challenges to a previous South Dakota informed consent law that required physicians read various state-mandated disclosures to patients prior to performing an abortion that included medically

inaccurate information about the risk factors of the procedure.[26] After initial challenges at the district court, in 2009 the Eight Circuit Court of Appeals ruled in *Planned Parenthood v. Rounds* that the portion of the informed consent law that required doctors disclose a link between abortion and an increased risk of suicide—a link rejected by nearly the entire medical community—was unconstitutional because it unduly burdened a pregnant person's right to chose abortion, in addition to violating doctors' First Amendment rights to be free from state-compelled speech.[27]

When rendering its decision, the court addressed this tension between mandated disclosures and medical standards of care, noting that common law duties of care that doctors owe patients already dictate what should and should not be disclosed in the course of treatment. Therefore, the specific requirements of the law that doctors disclose a heightened risk of suicide or suicide ideation was unnecessary.

But if medical standards of care made these specific state-mandated disclosures unnecessary, the fact that the medical community did not generally recognize a causal connection between suicide and abortion made the risk of misleading pregnant patients out of getting an abortion very real. "Legislatures have 'wide discretion to pass legislation in areas where there is medical and scientific uncertainty,'" the court held, "but the suicide advisory asserts certainty on the issue of medical and scientific knowledge where none exists."[28] The court didn't stop there. "The required suicide advisory would significantly constrain doctors' exercise of their professional judgment. South Dakota common law already requires doctors to inform patients of all the known material or significant risks of a medical procedure.[29] Thus, if a doctor considers suicide a known material risk of abortion, there is a common law duty to warn patients. Doctors didn't need South Dakota legislators mandating what was already a common law duty.

It is the focus on whether the content of the statement is truthful that is important here. From the position of the state of South Dakota and the proponents of this early mandated disclosure, the connection between suicide ideation and risk was the truth, despite the fact that the professional medical community disagreed. In the battle of medical testimony, anti-abortion advocates came up short, according to the court:

> The record does not demonstrate a generally recognized causal connection between abortion and suicide. In fact, it reveals vigorous debate over whether an apparent statistical correlation results from common cofactors rather than a showing that one causes the other. In the course of evaluating relevant peer reviewed literature, the American Psychological Association concluded that there is no evidence that risk of mental health problems among women who abort unwanted pregnancies is any greater than that of women who miscarry or deliver such pregnancies.[30]

It was on this point that pro-choice advocates had scored a major victory. Despite the latitude an abortion-hostile Supreme Court had granted state legislatures in crafting anti-abortion regulations, they did not have license to lie. Or they didn't until July 24, 2012, when the Eighth Circuit Court of Appeals ruled that they did. In a decision that fully reversed that earlier victory, a panel of conservative justices all appointed by Ronald Reagan held that the suicide disclosure was, in effect, not a lie, and that doctors must tell patients they run an increased risk of suicide for having an abortion because that information will "help" them make an informed decision regarding their medical care.[31]

The *Rounds* battle over informed consent and compelled disclosure illustrates the very damaging effect of the *Gonzales* decision. When there is a battle over scientific evidence to support a proposed medical regulation like disclosure of an abortion-suicide link, state legislatures are free to choose which evidence they believe and courts must defer to that choice, even if there is a mountain of evidence to the contrary. "Based on the record, the studies submitted by the State are sufficiently reliable to support the truth of the proposition that the relative risk of suicide and suicide ideation is higher for women who abort their pregnancies compared to women who give birth or have not become pregnant," the *Rounds* ruling declared.[32] It didn't matter that the journal articles cited as evidence to support the alleged causation between abortion and suicide had been discredited by further research, or that no one had been able to replicate the original study's findings. In fact, the article was believed to be so fatally flawed that the journal that published it was considering retracting it altogether.[33] The Supreme Court in *Gonzales* had given the Eighth Circuit the cover it needed when it ruled that nothing prevented legislatures like South Dakota from coming up with new, stricter definitions of medical risk in the context of restricting access to abortion. And the Eighth Circuit took it.

Basically, the court ruled that in order to render the suicide advisory unconstitutionally misleading or irrelevant, Planned Parenthood would have had to show that abortion has been ruled out, to a degree of scientifically accepted certainty, as a statistically significant causal factor in post-abortion suicides. And Planned Parenthood would have to make this showing of "scientifically accepted certainty" despite the fact that a lack of such certainty is not required to justify the disclosure in the first place. Simply put, in South Dakota, when legislating against reproductive rights, abortion restrictions didn't need to be supported to a medical degree of certainty, but challenges to those restrictions did.

•

Even without taking effect in South Dakota, H.B. 1217 still had an influence on anti-abortion laws in other states. In May 2012, Utah decided to pass a similar seventy-two hour waiting period. The only difference was that Utah left out the requirement that a pregnant person visit a crisis pregnancy center for an evaluation during her wait. However, other than frustration that the state had added another hurdle to accessing abortion, or anger than the government was intruding on personal medical decisions, the Utah law had little effect. According to Heather Stringfellow, Vice President of Public Policy at the Planned Parenthood Action Council of Utah at the time, "the law really hasn't changed anything. We are still providing abortions in a similar number to what we were prior to the law. We don't see people not returning more often. Women still make their decisions before they come in for the consultation before the abortion. Most people just kind of take it in stride. There have been a handful of women and partners who have been very dismayed and upset by having to wait for three days. There have been a handful of people who have been pretty traumatized by the affair. But few people are surprised that there are all these hoops they have to jump through."[34]

Could the fact that the extended wait period had no effect on changing a patient's mind have supported the state of South Dakota's stance that H.B. 1217 did not represent an undue burden under *Casey*? That concern may have been behind Planned Parenthood's decision to discontinue their full challenge of the bill. In December, 2012, Sarah Stoesz, President and CEO of Planned Parenthood Minnesota, North Dakota South Dakota announced that the organization would request that their challenge to the seventy-two-hour waiting period associated with the bill be dropped, choosing to focus more resources on the mandatory crisis pregnancy center visit portion of the bill. "Currently, we are focusing our energy and resources on fighting the most egregious part of this law—the

Crisis Pregnancy Center requirement," Stoesz said in a released statement. "We still believe the 72-hour waiting period provision of this law is unconstitutional and an example of politicians interfering in the medical care of women. However, we have found a way to implement this provision while minimizing the negative effects for our patients." [35] Planned Parenthood asked for the challenge to be dropped "with prejudice," meaning that they would reserve the right to challenge again down the road if circumstances changed.

South Dakota abortion opponents, meanwhile, didn't push the issue on the CPC requirement, but they still found a way to use the pretense of outside crisis pregnancy centers being needed to check for "coercion" prior to an abortion. In March of 2013, the Governor of South Dakota once again signed a waiting period bill—this time stating that weekends and holidays don't count as part of the three-day wait. Their reasoning? "[T]he law needs to be changed in case the counseling requirement takes effect," said bill sponsor John Hanson. "Counselors in pregnancy counseling centers might not be available on weekends and holidays, so the law should make sure centers have time to meet with women considering abortion." [36]

By dropping the challenge to the waiting period—and not the counseling portion of the law—Planned Parenthood didn't just open the gates for South Dakota to tweak their extended waiting period and make it even longer, but also provided abortion opponents with the precedent they needed to consider passing similar super-size waits in other low abortion access states. Two-day mandatory waiting periods requiring a pair of face to face clinic visits requirements became law in Arkansas, Alabama and Tennessee (although Tennessee's is currently blocked by a judge) while Missouri, North Carolina and Oklahoma all passed their own seventy-two-hour mandatory waiting periods—although neither North

Carolina nor Oklahoma made the initial appointment to begin the count-down be an in person visit.

The same was not true for Missouri, which, like North Dakota, has only one clinic in the state, making the mandatory three-day wait an excessive burden for those who are seeking out an abortion. Missouri legislators didn't view this to be much of a roadblock, comparing the need to wait for an abortion to be like thinking over major purchases for the home or family. "Even when I buy a new vehicle—this is my experience, again—I don't go right in there and say I want to buy that vehicle, and then, you know, you leave with it," Republican State Representative Chuck Gatschenberger said during testimony. "I have to look at it, get information about it, maybe drive it, you know, a lot of different things. Check prices. There's lots of things that I do, putting into a decision . . . Whether that's a car, whether that's a house, whether that's any major decision that I put in my life. Even carpeting. You know, I was just considering getting some carpeting or wood in my house. And that process probably took, you know, a month, because of just seeing all the aspects of it."[37]

The three-day waiting period easily passed Missouri's legislature in 2014, but was vetoed by Democratic Governor Jay Nixon, who opposed the lack of an exception for those impregnated by sexual assault. The veto was overridden, and the new bill went into effect. With the election of Republican Governor Eric Greitens in 2017, a special session was called to focus on the abortion issue, which included revamping the seventy-two-hour waiting period. Prior to this, patients seeking an abortion who didn't live near St. Louis, the site of the state's only clinic, could go to a local Planned Parenthood location to meet with a doctor for the "informed consent" information that kicked off the mandatory wait. This loophole eased the burden of travel time, childcare coverage or work hours lost for those who were trying to end an unwanted pregnancy, since an actual trip to St. Louis would only be required once during the process.

A proposed new bill would change the requirement to ensure that the patient must see the same doctor at each appointment, even though the information—a boilerplate pamphlet of "Women's Right to Know" data regarding fetal development, agencies that offered care if a person wanted to continue their pregnancy, ways to get child support from an unwilling partner, and of course medically inaccurate and unproven tidbits about the health risks and long-term consequences of having an abortion—was the same no matter who provided it or where it was offered.

That mandate that all patients must go to the St. Louis Planned Parenthood clinic—and no other healthcare agency in the state—twice and in person in order to terminate a pregnancy passed in October 2017, and remains in effect. Meanwhile, Governor Greitens, the anti-abortion hero who called the special session, was forced to resign seven months later over a sex scandal involving alleged blackmail of a former sex partner.[38]

In the end, perhaps the greatest irony is that all of these mandatory waiting periods— which include face-to-face doctor visits, pamphlets with medically discredited "abortion facts" (often an ultrasound with fetal or embryonic description and the playing of a heartbeat), and a "cooling off" period to go home and rethink the abortion—are supposedly done with the intention of stopping "coerced abortions." Yet, the most coercive factor when it comes to having an abortion is actually the state legislatures and their laws.

8

WASHINGTON, DC

TUG OF WAR, MEDICAID-STYLE

As a quirk of being the nation's capitol, Washington, DC has little control over its own budget and laws, and what control it does have is granted by the US Congress. However, when James Madison decided that Congress should have ultimate decision-making power when it came to legislating on the city's behalf, he likely never realized what a coup it would become for those who want to limit access to a full spectrum of reproductive health care services.

The fight over abortion rights reached a fever pitch in Washington, DC in 2012, when the US House of Representatives proposed numerous bills that would directly affect abortion laws in the city. In essence, conservative legislators decided to treat the city as a microcosm of what abortion opponents wanted to do across the country. The most controversial bill was Arizona representative Trent Franks's attempt to block the city from allowing any abortions after the fetus reached twenty weeks—a version of the 2010 "fetal pain" bill that had been passed in Nebraska. Since no one had challenged the Nebraska law, and it had passed in other states,

Franks believed that it was a constitutionally sound law that should also be passed in DC, too.[1]

Abortion rights advocates and medical professionals disagreed. DC's congressional delegate, Eleanor Holmes Norton, argued that if the bill were so sound, Franks and his cohorts should pass a federal version instead. "Why wouldn't they put this bill in for the entire country if they feel so deeply about it?" Norton asked the *Huffington Post*. "The reason is that they're bullies, so they know that you pick on the district whose member cannot vote on the House floor, you pick on the member who does not have any senators to protect her, and maybe you can get somewhere."[2]

It seemed Holmes had a point, as Franks had proposed the same restrictions when he was in the Arizona House of Representatives in the mid-1980s, which had failed to pass. Gloria Feldt, the former president of Planned Parenthood, recalled that it was the constant pressure from women's rights activists in the state that had kept Franks's attempts to limit abortion restrictions in check. "In Arizona we had done things like defeating a ballot initiative that would have outlawed most abortions, all except rape and incest, by the largest percentage that has ever happened to defeat a ballot initiative in the state," Feldt recalled. "We had gotten rid of Trent Franks, who is now back in Congress proposing the same legislation that he tried to get passed in Arizona that he couldn't."[3] Abortion activists were just as anxious to keep Franks in check in DC, but without the ability to vote him out of office, it was hard to have much impact.

•

The right to an abortion has been a tug-of-war issue ever since *Roe v. Wade* was passed in 1973, especially for those who are poor and lack health insurance, a group that disproportionally includes people of color.

In many ways, Washington, DC is an ideal barometer of this back-and-forth. For the past four decades, whenever the Republican Party has had control of the House of Representatives, it has voted to ban Washington, DC from using Medicaid funds to pay for abortions for pregnant people in poverty. When Democrats regain control of the House, the ban is repealed, and Medicaid abortions are allowed again. This pattern continued into the Obama administration. In July 2009, because Democrats controlled the White House, Senate and House, Washington, DC was allowed to use its own Medicaid funding to assist low-income patients in obtaining abortions.

Marcia D. Greenberger, founder of the National Women's Law Center, explained that allowing DC to fund abortions for the poor is a matter of social justice and equality. "Restrictions on public funding for abortion disproportionately affect women of color, a quarter of whom in DC are living in poverty and are more likely to rely on public funding for basic medical services," Greenberger said. "The time needed to save money, if indeed they even can, often results in poor women experiencing delays in obtaining an abortion. The greater the delay in obtaining an abortion, the less safe the procedure becomes. Those women who are unable to secure the funds can be denied affordable services altogether."[4]

Following the 2010 midterm elections, Democrats lost their majority in the House and the DC Medicaid abortion funding ban returned.[5] This time the ban was reinstated as a condition in last-minute negotiations to prevent a potential government shutdown caused by a congressional impasse over a new budget. House Republicans, feeling emboldened by their transition from minority to majority, as well as a wave of victories across the country that had turned multiple legislative bodies and even entire states to Republican control, roadblocked the passage of a continuing resolution that would have provided additional funding for the daily operations of the government. Their original asking price to keep the government afloat was the complete elimination of all Title X family planning funding. In this case, the Democrats held strong and refused to allow money for contraceptives, health screenings and treatment for sexually transmitted infections to be eliminated, as this would have left the poor without quality care. The House Republicans then modified their request: they would leave in family planning for the poor in place for the rest of the country, but in exchange, Washington, DC would once again have to give up its local funding of abortion for patients who lacked financial means.

Congresswoman Norton tried to stop the ban before it could be enacted. Prior to the final deliberations, she sent a letter to President Obama urging him not to let the poor pregnant people of Washington, DC be used as pawns. "It would be unacceptable to use the District's low income women as a bargaining chip at a time when women's rights advocates and the District have been particularly focused on protecting the city from a return to this restriction," she wrote. "District residents, women's rights advocates and the entire civil rights community worked too hard to remove all DC riders while Democrats controlled Congress to have their efforts immediately turned around at the insistence of House Republicans."[6] However, the president and congressional Democrats yielded to the Republicans and the ban was put back in place as part of the final continuing resolution budget deal passed on April 8, 2011. Norton was livid. "It looks to me that we were easy enough to throw under a bus, and that's where we landed," she told the *New York Times.* "The district becomes a sitting duck."[7]

The clinics that had previously scheduled procedures were surprised to learn that the ban was going into effect immediately and that as of Wednesday, April 13, at midnight, Medicaid would no longer cover terminations. "Tonight we received an urgent call from a partner clinic to notify us that DC Medicaid is ending its coverage of abortions at MIDNIGHT TONIGHT," the DC Abortion Fund (DCAF) wrote on its webpage. "The clinic had to call 28 women who are scheduled tomorrow and bringing their DC Medicaid as payment that they need to fundraise for the total cost of their procedure by their appointment tomorrow because Medicaid will no longer cover the cost of their abortion. These women are devastated."

Val Vilott, who at the time was the board president of DCAF, vividly remembers the panicked call she received from the clinic once it learned that insurance would no longer cover the remaining payments for the more than two dozen pregnant people who would be having second-trimester terminations the following morning. The total cost was likely to run $1500 per patient. "The clinic was trying to find out if they needed to tell these women to reschedule or if they could raise the money," recalled Vilott. "Postponing the procedure would mean that the cost would go up. The cost was already a barrier for these women, and now it was about to become an increasingly tall one."[8]

The DCAF board took an emergency vote and agreed to cover the difference between the cost of the abortions and what the scheduled patients could afford to pay. As a result, DCAF had to fundraise to try to regain the emergency funding it had provided. "We needed to combat the hit to our own finances," explained Vilott. "To fund twenty-eight patients in one day is not something that is typically a part of our process. Normally we have a very strict and regimented budget that we work with and per-patient caps based on the term of the pregnancy. This broke away from our system altogether." With the help of its email and social networks, DCAF was able to raise the money it needed to recoup the costs of the last-minute blow to its already stretched budget. But although those twenty-eight patients were able to have their procedures, other pregnant people who planned to use Medicaid to pay for their abortions were left on their own financially.

•

Only fifteen states in the country currently allow Medicaid to pay for abortions in most instances, rather than just in cases of rape, incest, or medical necessity (or, in the case of South Dakota, only if the patient's life is in jeopardy—there is no exception for a patient pregnant due to sexual assault).[9] For those states, allowing terminations to be covered by Medicaid is a civil rights issue. In Minnesota, for example, the State Supreme Court ruled in 1995 in the case of *Doe v. Gomez* that since a person has a legal right to an abortion, abortion services must be paid for via Medicaid in situations where the patient doesn't have the money to pay for the termination. The *Doe* ruling stated that a pregnant person does not lose access to abortion simply because they don't have the ability to pay for one. Otherwise, abortion is a right only for those who aren't poor. Megan Peterson, the former president of the National Network of Abortion Funds (NNAF), explained the problems many people have obtaining enough money to have an abortion in states with a funding ban: "As we know from other states where Medicaid doesn't cover abortions, it basically means that women don't get the abortions they need or want, or they go to great lengths and endure significant hardship in order to come up with the money."[10]

The average first-trimester abortion, be it medication or surgical, costs about $500 out of pocket. Add on to that additional expenses, such as for gas to travel back and forth to appointments and to adhere to waiting periods, lodging if the provider is too far away for the patient to do a round trip easily in one day, childcare for the 60 percent of patients seeking abortions who already have children, and time away from work for those who are employed. According to the Guttmacher Institute, which tracks research and trends in reproductive health care:

> In 2008, just one-third of privately insured U.S. women having abortions used that coverage to pay for their procedures; it is not clear how many of their plans offered full or partial coverage for abortion, or how many women were deterred from using their coverage because of concerns about confidentiality. Among women having abortions that year, methods of payment included paid out of pocket (almost 60%), private insurance (12%), and Medicaid (20%; almost all of whom lived in the few states that use their own funds to cover medically necessary abortions).[11]

The problem of paying for abortion care has only grown worse since the passage of the Affordable Care Act. Once hoped to be a panacea of health care reform in the wake of greedy insurers and unequal and discriminatory coverage procedures, the ACA—i.e, Obamacare—became bogged down by anti-abortion and anti-birth control interests on the right even before its passage. In an effort to obtain the last few votes needed in the House, the final version of the bill included the Stupak amendment—named after Michigan Democrat and abortion opponent Bart Stupak—which banned federal funding of abortion in the healthcare plans available on the insurance exchanges, since those plans would be getting tax credits and other government subsidies. The language was also added to the Senate version to woo Nebraska's Democratic Senator Mike Nelson, another abortion foe.

The language did more than just allow states to ban insurance policies purchased on the federal exchange from covering abortions—something that twenty-six states in the nation chose to do: it also allowed states to ban private insurance companies from offering abortion coverage as well. As a work around for the companies that wanted to allow private insurance coverage of abortion, the Stupak amendment opened the door for so-called "riders" to be offered so those who wanted to still have abortion coverage in their private health insurance plans could pay a separate premium in order to keep that care. Today, nine states claim to offer abortion coverage in a separate rider, yet not one of those states appears to actually be following through.[12]

Even more potentially devastating is the impact the policy could have on states that do mandate insurance coverage for abortion care. In California, one of the few states that requires that an insurance plan that covers prenatal costs and delivery must also cover abortion expenses, a new procedure being introduced by the Trump administration will require any insurer that is subsidized by public funds to send a second, separate bill to every enrollee in the insurance program, asking for one additional dollar to pay for their abortion coverage. The actual process of sending out, tracking and processing the payments are of course expected to cost far more than the funds being brought in, and will damage the state's health care system in total as a result.[13]

Of course, that's exactly the point.

•

So how do pregnant people pay for abortions and the associated expenses, which can easily come to $1000 just for a first-trimester procedure, especially those who are struggling financially (which is among the primary reasons women choose not to continue their pregnancies in the first place)? It's a question the National Network of Abortion Funds is often asked, and one for which they have developed an extensive list of answers. "Abortion funds may be able to help you pay for your abortion and you may be able to get a discount at your clinic," the group's website says. "But abortion funds just don't have the money to cover the entire cost of your abortion, so you're going to need to come up with some money on your own."[14] Unfortunately, most of the ideas the organization suggests will either drive a person farther into debt or force them to accept someone else's generosity simply in order to control their own reproductive freedom. Advice includes: cashing in bonds and returning recently purchased items to stores for cash; selling gift cards at less than face value; selling belongings; and borrowing money from friends, family or support groups. For those who don't want to explain to others what the funding is needed for, the group suggests financing the abortion with money meant to pay other bills and then asking friends or family members for a loan to pay those bills.

Raising the money to pay for an abortion also takes time for most people, and the farther along the gestational age, the more expensive the termination becomes. After ten weeks gestation, a medication abortion is no longer an option; after about fourteen weeks gestation, many states won't perform an abortion in a clinic, requiring patients to go to hospitals or travel to other states. With each delay comes a new expense; each new expense creates another delay. For some the delays accumulate to the point that they can no longer have an abortion at all. "The research literature clearly shows that restricting Medicaid funding for abortion forces many poor women— already at greatest risk of unintended pregnancy—to carry an unwanted pregnancy to term," reported Dr. Stanley Henshaw, a senior fellow at the Guttmacher Institute and author of the 2009 study *Restrictions on Medicaid Funding for Abortions: A Literature Review.* "Antiabortion advocates are using these restrictions in a misguided attempt to reduce the nation's abortion rate. Instead, we should be focusing on reducing the underlying cause of abortion—unintended pregnancy—by ensuring better access to and use of contraceptives." According to Henshaw's research, low income people who do not have access to abortion coverage via Medicaid tend to delay their abortions an average of two to three weeks as they try to come up with the money to pay. In the end, approximately 25 percent of low income patients seeking abortions are forced to give birth because funding for a termination is unavailable.[15]

That average is consistent with what Val Vilott saw at DCAF. "They just disappear," she said, referring to those who start the process of trying to get an abortion but eventually give up because there are too many barriers. "There is a continual kind of drop-off as the process goes on . . . We never know whether something came up, whether they got called in to work, whether a partner found out and they suddenly don't feel comfortable—we have no way of knowing that. We are very conscientious about racing the clock." It's a race that many lower-income pregnant people seeking help in order to afford a termination lose. "Women who are good advocates for themselves still aren't able to come up with hundreds and hundreds of dollars to help cover that procedure." For these people, there is no "equal access" to health care, and there may never be.

•

It took the Supreme Court less than a decade following the *Roe* decision in 1973 to pivot from finding that a person had a liberty interest in being free from coerced procreation, to endorsing the ability of states to regulate that interest out of existence by banning the use of Medicaid dollars to pay for abortions.

Title XIX of the Social Security Act established the Medicaid program, under which participating states could provide federally funded medical assistance to persons in need. The statute required states to provide qualified individuals with financial assistance in five general categories of medical treatment, including inpatient and outpatient hospital and physicians' services.[16] Although Title XIX did not require states to provide funding for all medical treatment falling within the five general categories, it did mandate that state Medicaid plans establish "reasonable standards" in delineating care available under Medicaid programs, so long as those services were "consistent with the objectives of [Title XIX]."[17]

The first funding challenge to reach the court came in 1977 and with it the embrace of a legal precedent for privileging state interests in "encouraging" childbirth over abortion. In the case of *Beal v. Doe*, a group of Medicaid-eligible pregnant women challenged a Pennsylvania regulation that prohibited the use of state Medicaid funds to pay for abortions for indigent women unless a physician certified in writing that the procedure was "medically necessary." The Pennsylvania regulation in effect at the time stated that an abortion was deemed "medically necessary," and therefore compensable under the state Medicaid program, if the pregnant person's health was at risk, if the fetus would be born with an incapacitating physical or mental deficiency, or if there was documented evidence that the pregnancy was a result of forcible rape or incest. If a physician certified that one of those conditions was met, then two other physicians would have to concur in writing and the procedure would have to be performed in a hospital.[18]

Among their claims, the plaintiffs in *Beal* alleged that Title XIX of the Social Security Act required Pennsylvania to provide coverage in its Medicaid plan for all abortions, not just those deemed "medically necessary." The plaintiffs objected to the exclusion of nontherapeutic abortions, or those that would not fit the definition of "medically necessary" from the state Medicaid program on both economic and health grounds. The former objection was based on the view that abortion is generally a less expensive medical procedure than childbirth. Therefore, states that refuse to fund nontherapeutic abortions are increasing public health costs, not reducing them.[19] Furthermore, the plaintiffs argued, banning nontherapeutic abortions also increased the risk to the pregnant patient, since early abortion poses less of a medical risk than childbirth.[20] The Supreme Court had already recognized pregnancy as a unique medical condition and therefore, the plaintiffs argued, the idea that it was reasonable for states to ban nontherapeutic—i.e., unnecessary—abortions should not apply.[21]

But the majority of justices on the court were not convinced by these arguments, and thus established by judicial fiat that low income pregnant people were not entitled to the same kind of access to abortion services as pregnant people with financial means. Without determining whether the plaintiffs' economic and health-related objections were accurate, the court did not agree that the exclusion of nontherapeutic abortions from Medicaid coverage was unreasonable under Title XIX. The plaintiffs, the court held, had failed to take into account the state's "valid and important interest in encouraging childbirth."[22] Although the court conceded that under *Roe*, before viability a person's constitutionally protected privacy interest outweighed that state interest, the majority was quick to clarify that even pre-viability, the state's interest in a patient's pregnancy was "significant" and continued to be so throughout the course of the pregnancy.[23]

Writing for a six to three majority, Justice Lewis Powell concluded that the statute merely required that participating states provide financial assistance to broad categories of care, nothing more. That meant that so long as a state's plan included reasonable standards for determining eligibility, and so long as those standards were consistent with the objectives of Medicaid, they were free to place restrictions on coverage for abortion access because those restrictions would not interfere with Medicaid's goal, which was "to enable each State, as far as practicable, to furnish medical assistance to individuals whose income and resources are insufficient to meet the costs of necessary medical services."[24] And, as if sensing the looming battles ahead, the court made it clear that states that tried to exclude necessary medical treatment from their Medicaid plans would likely run afoul of Title XIX, whereas because these were "elective" abortions—what the court characterized as "unnecessary (though perhaps desirable) medical services"—excluding them was completely consistent with the Social Security Act.[25]

While Justices William J. Brennan, Thurgood Marshall and Harry Blackmun each filed separate dissents in the case, it was clear that not even five years after *Roe*, the retreat from reproductive rights as a matter of settled law had begun.

•

Beal wasn't the only funding challenge to appear before the Supreme Court in 1977. In the case of *Maher v. Roe*, a Connecticut regulation limited state Medicaid benefits for first-trimester abortions to those that were "medically necessary," a term that was defined to also include psychiatric necessity. (The state enforced a limitation on psychiatric necessity by requiring prior authorization from the Department of Social Services before an abortion could be performed.) In order to obtain authorization for a first-trimester abortion, the hospital or clinic where the abortion was to be performed had to submit, among other things, a certificate from the patient's attending physician stating that the abortion was medically necessary. Two indigent women who were unable to obtain this certificate challenged the regulation, contending that Title XIX of the Social Security Act required the state of Connecticut to provide coverage in its Medicaid plan for all abortions, not just those that were medically necessary. The plaintiffs claimed that Connecticut had to treat abortion and childbirth equally in its regulation and couldn't show a policy preference by funding only medical expenses related to childbirth.[26] The plaintiffs also challenged the funding restrictions on equal protection grounds, arguing that it was discriminatory for the state to prefer childbirth over abortion in funding.

Again by a six to three vote, the Supreme Court held that the Constitution did not require states to pay for the costs of nontherapeutic abortions for indigent patients. Writing for the majority a second time, Justice Powell pointed out that the Constitution "imposes no obligation on the States to pay the pregnancy-related medical expenses of indigent women, or indeed to pay any of the medical expenses of indigents."[27] However, he added, "when a State decides to alleviate some of the hardships of poverty by providing medical care, the manner in which it dispenses benefits is subject to constitutional limitations."[28]

For purposes of equal protection analysis, a statute, regulation or policy is subject to "strict scrutiny" if it classifies on the basis of a suspect personal characteristic (e.g., race, national origin, alienage) or if it impinges on the exercise of a fundamental constitutional right. In this case, the court determined that the Connecticut abortion funding limitation did neither. "An indigent woman desiring an abortion does not come within the limited category of disadvantaged classes so recognized by our cases," Powell wrote.[29] "Nor does the fact that the impact of the regulation falls upon those who cannot pay lead to a different conclusion," because the court "has never held that financial need alone identifies a suspect class for purposes of equal protection analysis."[30] Furthermore, the court held, a poor person wasn't really injured by the privilege accorded to pregnancy by the Connecticut statute because they were no worse off than if the state had chosen not to favor childbirth, since it already prevented Medicaid funds for nontherapeutic abortions.

Having decided that the regulation limiting abortion funding did not require application of the strict scrutiny standard of review, the most rigorous legal test a court can apply when considering the constitutionality of a law regulating a personal right, the court then considered whether the limitation satisfied the more relaxed rational basis standard of review. Under that standard, the question was whether the distinction the regulation drew between childbirth and nontherapeutic abortion was "rationally related" to a "constitutionally permissible" purpose.[31] The court concluded that it was. "*Roe* itself," Justice Powell observed, "explicitly acknowledged the State's strong interest in protecting the potential life of the fetus . . . an interest honored over the centuries."[32] The Connecticut regulation "rationally furthers that interest," Justice Powell explained, because "the medical costs associated with childbirth are substantial" and "significantly greater than those normally associated with elective abortions during the first trimester."[33] Subsidizing the costs incident to childbirth "is a rational means of encouraging childbirth," he concluded.[34]

Justice Brennan, joined by Justices Marshall and Blackmun, dissented and cut right to the chase, namely that the court's decision would force poor people to carry unwanted and dangerous pregnancies to term. "As a practical matter," Brennan wrote, "many indigent women will feel they have no choice but to carry their pregnancies to term because the State will pay for the associated medical services, even though they would have chosen to have abortions if the State had also provided funds for that procedure, or indeed if the State had provided funds for neither procedure."[35]

•

If states are free to restrict Medicaid funding for nontherapeutic abortions, what happens if federal funding for those that are permitted becomes unavailable? Are states required to step in? That was the issue before the court in *Harris v. McRae*. And the answer was no.

Almost immediately following the 1976 passage of the Hyde Amendment, which blocked Medicaid insurance from covering abortion except in very specific cases, the law faced a legal challenge in federal court in New York. Cora McRae, a New York Medicaid recipient, pressed her case that Hyde violated her Fifth Amendment due process rights as well as the First Amendment's establishment clause. On the day the lawsuit was filed, the federal court issued a nationwide injunction preventing implementation of the Hyde Amendment while the legal challenges proceeded. Months later, the Supreme Court decisions in *Beal v. Doe* and *Maher v. Roe*—establishing that states were not required to reimburse for elective abortions—effectively lifted the New York district court's injunction and sent the case back for reconsideration. The game was afoot.

Judge John Francis Dooling Jr., who handled the *McRae* case from the beginning, issued a temporary restraining order, thereby preventing the then named Department of Health, Education and Welfare from implementing the law and temporarily protecting the rights of the poor to more broadly access abortions. But, on June 30, 1980, in *Harris v. McRae*, a sharply divided Supreme Court reversed Judge Dooling's order and held that the extreme limitations on Medicaid funding in the Hyde Amendment were constitutional. The court had approved the elimination of abortion from publicly funded health care programs even in cases where a pregnant person's health was gravely endangered or if they were pregnant as a result of rape or incest. The decision was nothing short of an affront to the foundations of *Roe* and an endorsement of segregating health care.

Under the Medicaid program, states were not obligated to fund abortions for which no federal funds were available. The court concluded that the Medicaid statute created a cooperative funding scheme and that if the federal government declined payment, the state did not have to provide the funds. Put another way, *Roe v. Wade* created no affirmative right to a government-funded abortion. Thus, it is permissible, the court said, for the government to use its funding powers to show a preference for childbirth over abortion.

Justice Brennan, joined by Justices Marshall and Blackmun, again led the dissent, finding that the denial of federal funding under the Hyde Amendment was tantamount to governmental coercion because it discouraged the poor and especially communities of color from exercising their abortion rights granted by *Roe*. Justice Marshall filed a separate dissent, finding that the denial of funding for abortions for the poor was "equivalent" to a denial of legal abortion. He said in this case the governmental benefit in the form of funding was vital because, barred from accessing service, a person would either seek an illegal abortion or carry a child to term and lose control over the direction of her life. Marshall wrote that the class of poor affected by the Hyde Amendment included many minorities and that the governmental interest at issue—the protection of potential life—did not measure up to the rights of the pregnant person. He predicted that decision would have a "devastating" impact on the lives and health of low income and minority communities. He couldn't have been more correct.

•

On the same day in 1980, the Supreme Court issued a companion ruling on the funding of abortion in *Williams v. Zbaraz*. This case involved an Illinois law that prohibited the use of state medical assistance funds to pay for abortions for indigent women under the state Medicaid program (and two other medical assistance programs financed solely with state funds) unless the procedure was necessary to preserve the life of the pregnant person. Two Illinois physicians who performed abortions, an indigent woman who alleged that she sought an abortion that was medically necessary but not necessary to save her life, and a welfare rights organization brought a lawsuit in federal district court challenging the funding restrictions.

The case bounced back and forth several times between the district court and the court of appeals, with the district court eventually holding that both the Hyde Amendment and the Illinois law denied indigent people seeking abortions equal protection under the law because each prohibited funding of "medically necessary abortions" even though all other medically necessary operations were funded.[36] Accordingly, both the state law and the Hyde Amendment were declared unconstitutional. The district court, however, enjoined enforcement only of the state law, not the Hyde Amendment. Under the law in effect at the time, the district court's judgment was appealed directly to the Supreme Court, bypassing the court of appeals.

In the first part of its opinion, the Supreme Court held that the district court lacked jurisdiction to decide the constitutionality of the Hyde Amendment because it had not been challenged by the plaintiffs, and thus vacated that portion of the lower court's judgment. In the second part of its opinion, the court noted that both plaintiffs' statutory claim (under Title XIX) and their constitutional claim (under the Equal Protection Clause) were foreclosed by the court's decision the same day in *Harris v. McRae*.[37] With that, the Supreme Court had conscribed poor women to a life where reproductive health services were not readily available and accessible.

•

How large a problem is the financial burden of paying for an abortion? In 2008, 40 percent of all abortions were obtained by people who were at or below the poverty level, according to the Guttmacher Institute; that rate had increased to nearly 50 percent by 2014.[38] While the rate of abortions in general was decreasing, thanks in part to greater access to contraception and sex education, for poor women, the number continued to grow.

The stories people tell about trying to find the money to afford the procedure can be heart-wrenching. On its website, Women's Medical Fund, an organization that helps provide funding to women in Pennsylvania who need abortions, tells the stories of a few of the women they have assisted:

> WS is the young mother of two small children. She supports her family on her monthly Social Security check of $670. She was sexually assaulted by her cousin and became pregnant from the rape. When he threatened to kill her if she told anyone about it, she was too fearful to turn to family members for help paying for her abortion. She managed to set aside some money from her monthly benefit check and $122 from WMF filled the remaining gap.

> PT is the young mother of a toddler who receives $158 per month in welfare to supplement her monthly wages of $140. Unable to afford her own place, she pays $150 each month to rent a room from a friend. Although she uses Medicaid for her other health care needs, she is prohibited from using it for an abortion. She struggled to set aside $200 toward the cost of her abortion, but her drug-addicted sister stole the money from her purse. After the theft, she turned to her mother and friends to borrow money, and WMF closed the gap with $96.

When seventeen-year-old BR's mother fell behind in the rent, the landlord evicted BR and her family from their apartment. She, her mother, and her 3 siblings moved into a motel room while her mother tried to come up with enough money for alternative housing. BR's boyfriend stopped returning her calls when she told him that she was pregnant. She is contributing her family's savings of $260 toward her abortion. WMF closed her gap with $210.[39]

In addition to these cases, there are also special situations in which even the pregnant person's health is affected by Medicaid abortion bans. In June 2012, the New York Abortion Access Fund sent out an emergency appeal on behalf of a woman they called "Sophia," who was being treated with chemotherapy for cancer and had been told that because of the treatment she would not be able to get pregnant. However, she did get pregnant, but because of the chemotherapy drugs the fetus suffered severe anomalies. Sophia was already too far along in her pregnancy for doctors in most states to be able to perform a termination, and in her state, Medicaid did not pay for abortion even when the mother was ill and the fetus was deemed incompatible with life.

There was just one clinic in the country able to perform the termination, but the cost was $12,000. Donors were stepping in, and the clinic offered to absorb as much of the cost as it could, but Sophia was still short nearly $2000. "It is clear that this young woman deserves our funding, yet $1750 is ten times our average grant amount," the fund wrote in a plea for help. "We are turning to you today to request an emergency contribution to help this woman terminate this pregnancy that poses serious risk to her health."[40] The fund did eventually receive the money it needed to help Sophia. However, as more people find it impossible to afford a termination, and more states refuse to allow them to use Medicaid to cover the cost of terminating a pregnancy, abortion funds have taken over the lion's share of filling in the gap, which is not a sustainable long-term solution.

By allowing Medicaid funding to pay for prenatal care and birthing costs but not for terminations, the government is essentially advocating for low income communities to give birth, regardless of their personal choice, a fate that others can avoid simply because they have the financial means. That was the argument behind a law in Washington State that would have required insurance plans to include coverage for abortion if they also covered maternity care. But when state Democrats tried to expand the scope of the bill to include both public and private insurance plans, Republicans killed it by tying it to the state's budget bill to block it from getting to the Senate for a vote.[41] It took nearly six years for the bill—eventually known as the Reproductive Parity Act—to finally make it through both chambers and get signed into law. Despite this, abortion opponents continue to oppose the bill by claiming it forces them as taxpayers or employers to violate their religious beliefs by "subsidizing abortion" and birth control.[42]

As frustrating as it is when anti-abortion politicians block legislation that would make it possible for those who are poor to have the same reproductive choices as people of means, at least pregnant people who live in states that deny coverage are being blocked by their own legislators. The same can't be said for those who reside in Washington, DC, where the preference of the majority of the residents is overruled by a group of lawmakers whom the citizens have no ability to hold responsible for their votes. This is why the House GOP choose Washington, DC as the arena for flexing their anti-abortion muscles.

Despite the fact that she quite literally had no voice, Congresswoman Eleanor Holmes Norton continued to advocate passionately on behalf of her constituents during that 2011 abortion insurance coverage battle, even if the media was her only audience. "During the past four years, I worked to carry out the will of DC residents and our local government by successfully removing all of the accumulated appropriations riders that eliminated the District's right to decide how to spend its local funds on behalf of its residents, including for abortion for low-income women," she said. "Not only do Republicans seek to trample on DC's rights as a self-governing jurisdiction, they apparently seek to trample on my right as a Member of Congress to participate in the legislative process by giving testimony on a bill that directly affects the District." Trent Franks and his anti-abortion cohorts might be relentless, but Norton swore she would be just as vigilant. "We will not give up on our efforts to use every legitimate means to stop all anti–home rule attempts to roll back the progress the District has made over the past four years, including today's attempt to prevent DC from funding abortions for low-income residents."[43]

Eight years later much has changed in Washington DC. President Barack Obama is gone, replaced by Republican Donald Trump. Arizona Senator Trent Franks is gone as well, resigning in 2017 after a scandal involving inappropriate interactions with his female staffers—including asking them if they would consider acting as surrogates for himself and his wife[44] What hasn't change, however, is the district's ability to regain Medicaid coverage for abortion procedures. And until the residents of Washington DC are allowed to have home rule—rather than Congress making decisions for them without their consent—the odds are they never will.

9

TEXAS

A BLUEPRINT FOR DEFUNDING
PLANNED PARENTHOOD

"I've met too many prospective moms and dads from all across Texas who want nothing more than the chance to love a child they can call their own. I know of too many families that have been blessed and made whole by the glorious gift of adoption to ever believe there can ever be such a thing as an 'unwanted child.'"[1] When Rick Perry, then serving as the Republican governor of Texas, spoke those worlds at a fundraiser for the Downtown Pregnancy Center of Dallas in 2009, he was celebrating the impact that organizations which supported women and teens who chose to carry pregnancies to term provided in the state.

That praise was well deserved. Between his gutting of family planning funding and his ceaseless vendetta against the state's Planned Parenthood affiliates, Perry was Texas's biggest roadblock to affordable contraception—especially for those who were uninsured, lacked contraception coverage, or relied on the state's low income Medicaid coverage to meet their health care needs.

Texas isn't the only state to use those on Medicaid as pawns in an attempt to cut off Title X family planning funding to Planned Parenthood. In 2011, Shelby County in Tennessee shifted its funding to Christ Community Health Services (CCHS), effectively cutting off Planned Parenthood Greater Memphis Region from Title X funds. While CCHS did not provide access to emergency contraception, or even provide referrals to places that did, it did offer a lecture on God. One patient testified at a public hearing that a practitioner told her, "If only my relationships with people and God were right, I would have fewer health problems."[2]

In response to Shelby County's action, in 2012, the federal government awarded Planned Parenthood Greater Memphis a three-year grant worth $395,000 annually for Title X family planning services. "This grant award means that Planned Parenthood will be able to resume providing essential health care services to the low income women and teens who depend us every day to help them plan their families, said PPGMR CEO Barry Chase said when the grant was announced. "It means our patients who qualify will be able to get the confidential, unbiased care they need from the provider they prefer and trust."[3]

While Tennessee tried to defund Planned Parenthood by choosing a different provider, Ohio attempted to defund the group by creating a hierarchy of providers that could have Title X funding, and put Planned Parenthood in last place on that list. The move was meant to ensure that funding would run out before Planned Parenthood ever got to the front of the line. Under the amendment, all family planning dollars in the state would first be allocated to local health departments, then "federally qualified community health centers [FQCHs]," a definition that didn't include Planned Parenthood clinics. Anything still left would go to private care centers, and, finally, Planned Parenthood. Advocating for this was Mike Gonidakas of Ohio Right to Life, who told the *Cleveland Plain Dealer* that family planning funding should be going to places like Lower Lights

Ministries, which also catered to low-income women. "This money should be going to them, as opposed to the abortion industry," Gonidakas said, either not knowing or not caring that the faith-based clinic he was referencing had multiple doctors who wouldn't even provide birth control.[4]

The amendment to reprioritize family planning funding in Ohio was added to the 2011 mid-budget review, but was stripped out after too much negative feedback from constituents. It was returned during the lame duck session in 2012, but Ohio State Senator Tom Niehaus refused to let that bill—or the contentious Heartbeat Ban—out for a vote. Gonidakas, meanwhile, was appointed to the State Medical Board, despite having no actual experience as a medical practitioner.

•

The Texas bid to defund Planned Parenthood wasn't any more popular with state residents than the Ohio effort was. The state was already deep in a healthcare crisis; less than half of its population had private insurance coverage, and a full quarter of its population was completely uninsured. In 2010, when the initial push to defund Planned Parenthood began, Texas ranked number one in the percentage of uninsured adults in the country, with nearly 5 million uninsured between the ages of 19 and 64.[5] The numbers were even worse for minority groups, as "37 percent of Hispanics/ Latinos, 21.4 percent of African Americans, and 21.1 percent of Asians" in state were uninsured, "compared to 13.5 percent of whites."[6] As a result, the state was suffering from an epidemic of adults who lacked primary care doctors and who often skipped preventative care all together, forced to use emergency rooms as their primary health care source.

The situation was even worse for anyone who got pregnant, especially the large Latina population in the state, who without access to a physician, would be unable to obtain birth control or other family planning needs, creating an enhanced likelihood of an unintended pregnancy and a continuing cycle of poverty. "Latinas as it stands currently have the least amount of access to health insurance of any ethic group of women in the United States," Veronica Bayetti Flores, then Policy Research Specialist at the National Latina Institute for Reproductive Health, explained in 2012.[7] "Low income Latinas who would otherwise qualify for public assistance such as Medicaid or any other kinds of programs that are there to provide public assistance either don't qualify because, if they're immigrant Latinas, sometimes they're undocumented. So that would prevent them from qualifying from a number of different healthcare programs." In fact, according to Flores, sometimes it took getting pregnant just to get any health care at all. "Those are some of the places where undocumented women are actually able to get care when they're pregnant. It's a disturbing feeling for them that that's actually one of the only times that they're able to receive any care, when they're pregnant. It's a little bit insulting to be treated like a vessel, right? But that's the only time you're eligible for care."

It was these sorts of issues that had made Title X funding a federal program in the first place. With the federal government providing grants, those who were poor, uninsured or using Medicaid could obtain well-women exams, contraception, prenatal care and other basic health reproductive health care services without having a primary physician or skipping medical needs due to the cost. Access to contraception would reduce unplanned pregnancy, cutting health expenses associated with abortion or giving birth. According to a 2012 report from the Brookings Institute, for every dollar spent on contraception, taxpayers save $2 to $6.[8]

These were the types of arguments that went into creating Texas's Medicaid Women's Health Program (WHP). The program served 130,000 low income, uninsured reproductive-aged people in the state, allowing them to visit providers for family planning needs and health screenings for cancer, as well as testing for sexually transmitted infections. The funding was used entirely for these screenings and for providing contraception, and no clinic that participated—including the Planned Parenthood affiliates in the program—offered abortions.

Yet it was the specter of "fungible funding" that Perry and his cohorts used to pass a law forbidding Planned Parenthood affiliates from being a part of the WHP. "Planned Parenthoods across the country provide abortions, are affiliated with abortion providers, or refer women to abortion providers," the governor's spokesperson told the *New York Times* in March 2012.[9] Republican State Representative Wayne Christian agreed. "I don't think anybody is against providing health care for women. What we're opposed to are abortions . . . Planned Parenthood is the main organization that does abortions. So we kind of blend being anti-abortion with being anti-Planned Parenthood."[10] But, in actuality, they were against "providing health care for women," at least if that health care had anything to do with preventing pregnancy. When the *Texas Tribune* asked Christian in a video interview if it was a "war on birth control," he responded, "Of course it's a war on birth control, abortion, everything—that's what family planning is supposed to be about."[11]

To assist in the defunding process, Texas first dropped its two-year budget for family planning from $111 million to $38 million.[12] The elimination of two-thirds of its budget would cut services for about 300,000 patients and was projected to lead to 20,000 unwanted pregnancies that would cost the state about $230 million, according to the state's legislative budget board.[13]

Those who were familiar with Perry's record knew that this wasn't a money saving endeavor. In 2005, he had taken a swing at the state's family planning funding, transferring $10 million to Federally Qualified

Health Centers (FQHCs), community based clinics that could provide a full range of health care services, choosing to fund those clinics instead of Planned Parenthood or reproductive health centers. However, like Lower Lights Ministries in Ohio, clinics that were religiously-based may not have a full range of family planning services for women to use. According to reporter Jordan Smith, those funds may have gone to FQHC's, but that doesn't mean patients were served. Smith wrote in *The Nation* that for the first year, $2 million of that $10 million was returned to the state, unused. The FQHCs continued to return funds every year, and their cost per client was over $50 per client more than what Planned Parenthood spent.[14] Perry also took $5 million in family planning funding and gave it to crisis pregnancy centers directly, allowing the state's crisis pregnancy network to use taxpayer funding to counsel women with unintended pregnancies to give birth rather than choose an abortion. According to a report by the *Washington Independent*, almost all of the $7 million in funding the state's pregnancy centers received went to Christian-centric non-profit agencies.[15]

•

It didn't take long for the federal government to make it clear that Texas's move to cut Title X funding was unacceptable. President Barack Obama's Department of Health and Human Services warned the governor that purposefully ousting Planned Parenthood as a provider and prohibiting the health care organization from receiving Title X funds put the state in danger of losing all of its family planning funding. Still, Perry continued to insist that it was the Obama administration that was putting its political agenda over the rights and well-being of the state's poor and uninsured. In a March 8. 2012 op-ed, he wrote:

Why would the Obama administration take away access to health care for low-income Texas women? Because this administration puts funding for abortion providers and affiliates ahead of funding for women's cancer screenings and other preventive health care. Texas, operating under the direction of an overwhelming and bipartisan majority of legislators, prohibits abortion providers and affiliates like Planned Parenthood from receiving taxpayer money. Because Texas refuses to fund abortion providers and their affiliates, the federal government has announced that it will cancel the Women's Health Program. To me, this reflects a twisted set of values, not to mention a continued disregard for the basic concept of states' rights.[16]

Perry approved the ban on Planned Parenthood affiliates being used in the WHP, even if it meant the loss of federal funds. He vowed to replace the lost $30 million from the state's own budget. "I am directing you to begin working with legislative leadership to identify state funding to continue to provide these services, in full compliance with Texas law, should the Obama Administration make good on its threat to end the health care to these 100,000-plus women," Perry wrote in a public letter to Texas Health and Human Services Commissioner Tom Suehs. "Texans send a substantial amount of our tax dollars to Washington, DC, and it is unacceptable that the Obama Administration is denying Texas taxpayers the use of those dollars to fund this program, simply because of its pro-abortion agenda."[17]

Supporting Perry in his mission were the Catholic Bishops of Texas, who argued that ousting Planned Parenthood as a provider—despite the fact that the Texas clinics in question didn't offer abortion services—actually reinforced "comprehensive" reproductive health care. "There are only 44 Planned Parenthood locations in the Women's Health Program and many do not provide comprehensive health care—say, for example, mammograms or many common gynecological services—which are critical for women's health," the group said. "It is the Texas bishops' position that true women's health services should be separated from services that are not health care: namely, contraception, sterilization, and abortion. By insisting that the state of Texas cannot direct funds to thousands of providers statewide who offer true, comprehensive, women's healthcare—and instead require Medicaid funds go to prop up 44 Planned Parenthood clinics—the federal government risks removing preventative health care from hundreds of thousands of women in Texas."[18]

That the group referred to contraception as "not health care" is telling. The Texas program was supposed to primarily offer family planning services to low income patients, yet those who were advocating for a Planned Parenthood-exclusionary system—saying alternative providers should be used instead—were also admitting that they don't believe birth control should be offered at all. It was a variation of the same argument used to oppose the birth control mandate in the Affordable Care Act. "The bishops want contraception out of the Affordable Care Act entirely," explained Jon O'Brien, President of Catholics for Choice. "That would affect all Americans. And if you think that's the whole story, again you are wrong."[19] According to O'Brien, the fight against contraception was based on the bishop's desire to continue to get federal funding for charity work, while at the same time being allowed to adhere to and enforce their own set of rules on others. "They've carefully constructed a very bogus argument taken to the far extreme," he stated. It would take a few more years—and one major Supreme Court decision—to learn exactly how correct O'Brien was.

The bishops got their way, as in March 2012, the state of Texas began phasing out the WHP. The first trick was to find new providers for the tens of thousands of patients relying on Planned Parenthood clinics to provide their exams and family planning services. Perry touted the over 2500 doctors in the state as a primary reason why it would be just fine to move women away from Planned Parenthood services. However, as Texas-based journalist Andrea Grimes discovered in her own personal investigation, getting in to see one was a lot more complicated without insurance:

> Most places I telephoned did not provide reproductive health care and instead focused on providing low-income housing, job training and addiction-recovery programs. A homeless shelter on the FQHC list did tell me I could get a free pap smear if I could prove I was homeless. I then got sidetracked looking into something called Project Access, a low-cost program that helps uninsured people who don't qualify for Medicaid—but because I made more than about $20,000 last year as an unmarried woman without kids, I don't qualify for that, either. And the Texas Breast and Cervical Services, which is supposed to provide low-cost screenings for Texas women? It referred me to Planned Parenthood. So that was a no-go.[20]

The full switch to the Texas funded program wasn't expected to be complete until November 1, 2012—conveniently a few days before the 2012 election. But concerns grew as patients were told that as of May 1, they would no longer be able to use Planned Parenthood as their provider. Texas Planned Parenthood filed suit against the state on April 11, and on April 30, the Fifth Circuit Court of Appeals blocked the ban from going into effect, saying it was "likely unconstitutional because it bars [Planned Parenthood] from participating in the Women's Health Program based on their affiliation with legally and financially separate entities that engage in constitutionally protected conduct related to abortion."[21]

Perry and his administration appealed the ruling by reassessing how a provider for the program could be barred. Now, instead of just being associated with an "abortion provider," they also banned any group that so much as referred for or even mentioned abortions.[22] This essentially created a state gag rule that many medical providers feared would put their ability to assist patients in jeopardy. Collectively, the Texas Medical Association, Texas division of the American College of Obstetricians and Gynecologists, the Texas Association of Obstetricians and Gynecologists, the Texas Academy of Family Physicians and the Texas Pediatric Society sent a letter to the Department of State Health expressing their concerns about the law. "The relationship between patient and physician is based on trust and creates the physician's ethical obligations to place the patient's welfare above his or her own personal politics, self-interest and above obligations to other groups," wrote the organizations, which represented over 47,000 medical practitioners. Among other worries was that doctors might leave the program because of the new regulation, making an already precarious provider situation even worse.[23]

·

As Perry continued to fight the federal government over reproductive health care, an even bigger storm brewed. In 2012, the Supreme Court ruled that the Affordable Care Act, President Barack Obama's signature health care reform bill, was constitutional, and that states would need to begin to work with the government to extend Medicaid eligibility or be prepared to give up their expansion funding. For a state that relied heavily on Medicaid, the expansion would be a boon to Texas by cutting the costs of the uninsured on the state healthcare system. On principle, however, Perry—who was about to embark on a doomed quest to be the 2012 Republican presidential nominee—remained as stubbornly committed to rejecting the ACA funding as he was to rejecting funding to the Women's Health Care program. The governor announced:

> In the ObamaCare plan, the federal government sought to force the states to expand their Medicaid programs by—in the words of the Supreme Court—putting a gun to their heads. Now that the "gun to the head" has been removed, please relay this message to the President: I oppose both the expansion of Medicaid as provided in the Patient Protection and Affordable Care Act and the creation of a so-called "state" insurance exchange, because both represent brazen intrusions into the sovereignty of our state. I stand proudly with the growing chorus of governors who reject the PPACA power grab. Thank God and our nation's founders that we have the right to do so. Neither a "state" exchange nor the expansion of Medicaid under the Orwellian-named PPACA would result in better "patient protection" or in more "affordable care." What they would do is make Texas a mere appendage of the federal government when it comes to health care.[24]

The governor and presidential wannabee was ready to play political chicken with the 25 percent of population in his state that was uninsured, and the federal courts had given him an opening to do so.

•

Title X of the Public Health Services Act authorizes the Secretary of Health and Human Services (HHS) to make grants and contract with either public entities or nonpublic private entities to help establish and operate voluntary family planning projects that are supposed to offer a broad range of "acceptable and effective family planning methods and services."[25] Since its inception in 1970, the Act has been the target of anti-abortion (and anti-birth control) activists, despite the fact that Section 1008 specifies that none of the federal funds appropriated under Title X "shall be used in programs where abortion is a method of family planning."

Despite the specific statutory language that prevents Title X funds from going to programs that provide abortion care, activists on the right have consistently pushed challenges to the program as a means to end it all together. For example, in 1988, HHS issued regulations that, among others things, prohibited Title X family planning projects from engaging in abortion counseling or referrals, and required Title X projects to maintain a "objective integrity and independence from the prohibited abortion activities" by using separate facilities, personnel and accounting records designed to provide "clear and operational guidance" to grantees about how to "preserve the distinction between Title X programs and abortion as a means of family planning."[26]

Those regulations placed three conditions on the grant of federal funds for Title X projects: they could not provide abortion counseling or referrals; could only provide "preconceptional services"; and must refer every pregnant client "for appropriate prenatal and/or social services by furnishing a list of available providers that promote the welfare of mother and unborn child."[27] Under the regulations issued by HHS in 1988, the scope of gag on abortion counseling or referrals was wide. Title X projects were prohibited from even "indirectly" encouraging or promoting abortion, such as by weighing the list of referrals in favor of providers which perform abortions, by including on the list of referral providers those whose principal business was the provision of abortions, by excluding from the list any available providers who did not provide abortions, or by "steering" clients to providers who offered abortion as a method of family planning.[28] Title X projects were also expressly prohibited from referring a pregnant person to an abortion provider, even if that person directly asked for such a referral.[29]

The regulations also broadly prohibited a Title X project from engaging in activities that "encourage, promote or advocate abortion as a method of family planning."[30] Forbidden activities included lobbying for legislation that would increase the availability of abortion as a method of family planning, developing or disseminating materials advocating abortion as a method family planning, providing speakers to promote abortion as a method of family planning, using legal action to make abortion available in any way as a method of family planning and paying dues to any group that advocates abortion as a method of family planning as a substantial part of its activities.[31] With these changes, Title X projects now also had to be organized so that they were "physically and financially separate" from prohibited abortion activities.[32] The regulations provided a list of nonexclusive factors for the Secretary to consider in conducting a case-by-case determination of this "objective integrity and independence" standard such as the existence of separate accounting records and separate personnel, and the degree of physical separation of the project from facilities for prohibited activities.[33] In short, the changes were extensive and created a host of new regulatory burdens on family planning programs that had no correlation to the delivery of family planning care and, by their very design, make accessing family planning services by the poor even more difficult than it had been earlier under Medicaid.

Before the 1988 regulations went into effect, Title X grantees and physicians who supervised Title X funds filed several lawsuits in federal court. After working its way through the lower courts, the challenge made its way up for Supreme Court review, and by a vote of five-to-four, the Court upheld the challenged regulations, solidifying a bias against reproductive services as part and parcel of comprehensive family planning.[34] Chief Justice William Rehnquist wrote the majority opinion for the Court and laid out, in painstaking detail, the case against parity in health care services for all women, and rejecting the plaintiffs' argument that the regulations were not authorized by Title X.[35]

The plaintiffs also argued that the regulations violated the First Amendment because they impermissibly discriminated on the basis of viewpoint—prohibiting discussion about abortion but mandating information promoting childbirth.[36] The Court rejected this argument outright, saying that when the government appropriates public funds to establish a program, it is entitled to define the limits of that program even if that means funding some rights at the expense of others.[37]

The Court also rejected plaintiffs' alternative First Amendment claim that the regulations conditioned the receipt of Title X funding on the relinquishment of a constitutional right, namely the right to engage in abortion advocacy and counseling.[38] According to the Court, this claim fell short because the government was not denying a benefit to anyone, but was instead "simply insisting that public funds be spend for the purposes for which they were authorized."[39] In addition, the regulations did not force a Title X grantee to relinquish any abortion-related speech, but simply required that the grantee keep such activities "separate and distinct from Title X activities."[40] The regulations, the Court explained, were aimed at Title X projects, not Title X grantees—a distinction that was significant on paper but fell short in the reality of Title X administration.

•

The final word in abortion funding cases and the battle over federal-state cooperation, until the Affordable Care Act decision, was *Dalton v. LRFPS*, a 1996 decision that made it clear states would be given wide berth in regulating the economics of abortion access. In *Dalton*, a group of Arkansas Medicaid providers and physicians who performed abortions brought a lawsuit in federal district court challenging an amendment to the Arkansas Constitution which prohibited the use of state funds to pay for any abortion "except to save the mother's life." The basis of the plaintiffs' lawsuit was that the state funding prohibition conflicted with the Hyde Amendment. The case eventually made its way to the Supreme Court where despite its usual preference for federal pre-emption, this time the conservative Rehnquist court handed states broad power to ban the use of funds for abortions. In short, states only needed to comply with the contours of Hyde. Nothing more, nothing less.[41]

•

Then in June 2012, the balance of power between federal and state cooperative spending was upended. In *National Federation of Independent Business v. Sebelius*, the Supreme Court, for the first time, invalidated a condition on federal spending on the grounds that it coerced the states. The decision provided the perfect cover for the Perry administration and the charge against universal health care access envisioned in the Affordable Care Act, especially for those capable of becoming pregnant.

The Affordable Care Act represented an unusual expansion of access and equalizing of price that embraced a vision of gender equality in health care and demanded the private sector provide parity in coverage. For those who opposed expanding care for women, LGBTQ and non-binary people, what better place than Texas to reinforce the isolationist state's rights approach to reproductive health care and to create a stand-off with the federal government over access to it. After all, Texas was the only politically deep red state with a large enough population that by standing alone and apart from the Medicaid program, it could cause significant political impact across the country. If that happened to harm marginalized communities, especially those without insurance, in the meantime, so be it.

Harm them it did. Within a year of the initial family planning cuts instituted by the Perry administration, documents showed that sixty clinics across the state were forced to close.[42] Of those sixty clinics, only a dozen were run by Planned Parenthood, the anti-abortion right's original target. Federally qualified health centers began refusing new clients because they lacked the resources to deal with the increase in numbers, and in remote areas, thousands of patients started going without services of any type due to lack of money and access. "[I]n hoping to punish Planned Parenthood, politicians had gone too far, with devastating consequences for women's health," wrote Carolyn Jones in an article for the *Texas Observer*. "Lawmakers, they said, had thrown the 'baby out with the bath water.'"[43]

Despite the obvious harm that came from continuing its vendetta against Planned Parenthood as a family planning and sexual health services provider, the state of Texas still refused to change course. Perry decided not to seek another term as governor and was succeeded by his Attorney General, Republican Greg Abbott, who continued his predecessor's quest to cut off reproductive rights access in the state. Access to family planning services dwindled even further as new providers recruited by the state's leading anti-abortion activists' organizations were discovered to be wasting millions of dollars while serving just a handful of patients. Foremost among them was Heidi Group, a Christian non-profit founded by a former abortion clinic director named Carol Everett, who had found

God and left the industry. Everett was appointed to the committee that sought alternatives to Planned Parenthood by Abbott, and Heidi Group was awarded an initial $5.1 million for family planning and another $1.6 million from Healthy Texas Women for 2017. Instead of the 70,000 clients it pledged to serve, Heidi Group providers served a mere 3,300 patients—about 5 percent of their target. The state responded by decreasing their budget by almost $4 million, but the organization still received another $3.2 million for fiscal year 2019.[44]

While Planned Parenthood remained outside of the providers who could be funded by Texas's two alternative low income family planning and sexual healthcare programs, other groups that did provide health care and didn't offer abortion either also continued to feel a pinch. According to an investigation by the *Houston Chronicle*, numerous high performing, high volume health centers—located mostly in rural and immigrant communities—were running out of funds to care for their own patients even as Heidi Group and its partners frittered away their own bankrolls. Altogether, the impact was undeniable. In 2017, the most recent year for which full data was available, the state had served 100,000 fewer patients than it had in 2010, the last year before Perry decided to dismantle the system to remove Planned Parenthood. And they spent $35 million more in the process.[45]

Despite the clear inadequacies exposed by Texas's attempt to defund and replace Planned Parenthood—and the exponential effect it had on low income and marginalized communities, including immigrants and people of color—other conservative states hopped on the bandwagon, testing their own creative approaches to blocking their Planned Parenthood affiliates from receiving state funds. According to the Guttmacher Institute, before 2015, eleven states (including Texas and Ohio) had put in place some sort of restriction banning the health care organization from receiving funding for sexual healthcare work—ranging from family planning to HIV prevention, sex ed programs or more. Since 2015, that number has increased to fifteen successful state restrictions, with another nine attempted but held up by the courts.[46]

Of course, the courts are unlikely to save this funding for long. On March 12, 2019, the Sixth Circuit Court of Appeals finally ruled on Ohio's lingering defunding scheme that put Planned Parenthood at the bottom tier for receiving state funding. The court's decision? There was no constitutional issue with allowing the state to deny funding to Planned Parenthood, as long as the clinics as a whole were providing abortions, even if the funds themselves weren't going to any type of abortion support. The ruling was decided 11 to 6, and 4 of those 11 judges were appointees of President Donald Trump.[47]

•

With a growing list of case law that allowed states to broadly regulate health-care spending related to abortion, a new decision upheld in a major circuit court and, finally, the Roberts court embrace of the legal theory of "coercion" related to federal-state cooperative spending, states are now freer than ever to cut off federal spending to clinics for reproductive health care. And in Texas, that's exactly what they've done, and with the Fifth Circuit Court of Appeals blessing.[48] The state has literally succeeded in creating its own separate reproductive health care and family planning medical system based entirely on income, and like our history of segregated public benefits, there's not a shred of equality in it. And despite a laundry list of clear and harmful consequences to vulnerable communities, more states are eager to follow Texas's lead.

Ironically, now that the states have finally broken new ground in escalating their war on funding Planned Parenthood, their individual efforts may no longer even be required. On February 22, 2019, the Trump administration announced a new federal rule that would prohibit Planned Parenthood affiliates from fully participating in the Title X Family Planning provision program by barring any organization that provides or refers for abortions from receiving funds. The new rule is expected to block any clinic that offers abortions, as well as effectively "gag" non-abortion providing clinics from giving referrals to those who are pregnant and want to terminate. At the same time, the administration pledges to move family planning dollars not just to federally qualified health care centers, but also religiously-affiliated medical groups that in many cases may not offer any forms of hormonal contraception at all.[49] Advocates have challenged the Trump administration's efforts to roll back Title X in a series of lawsuits across the country, meaning that the increasingly conservative Supreme Court will likely have the final say.

10

KANSAS

ALWAYS LET YOUR CONSCIENCE BE YOUR GUIDE

In the Disney version of *Pinocchio*, Jiminy Cricket tries to keep the fumbling puppet on the straight and narrow path, telling the wooden boy that he should let his "conscience" tell him what to do. "When you get in trouble and you don't know right from wrong . . . Give a little whistle! And always let your conscience be your guide," Jiminy Cricket eagerly advises. It's a simple message that makes most decisions black or white, avoiding any potential gray areas and providing comfort in moral absolutism. This absolutism has been taken to its extreme in the state of Kansas, where conscience trumps all when it comes to decisions involving reproductive health and autonomy, no matter how tangentially the "provider" is involved.

Conscience clauses have long played a role in medicine, primarily in Catholic hospitals and health clinics, where doctors and nurses have refused to provide birth control or emergency contraception, offer sterilizations or terminate pregnancies. Meant to protect a religious medical provider from participating in something that could be viewed as a moral sin, conscience waivers reflected a paternalistic attitude that went hand in hand with the belief that women weren't able to make their own medical decisions, and needed a man—whether it be a husband, father or religious advisor—to provide guidance and permission.

These clauses were originally seen as protecting the individual rights of people affiliated with religious institutions, but as anti-abortion advocates ramped up their fight on choice over the past several decades, these clauses expanded to allow entire corporate health care systems to refuse to supply services or abide by non-discrimination policies that conflict with their religious beliefs. As religiously-affiliated groups and Catholic hospitals in particular have taken over larger portions of the health care system, as well as a greater share of the clinics that provide day to day and preventative care for lower income and uninsured individuals, religious doctrine and dogma have created serious roadblocks to patient care and safety. For example, many Catholic hospitals refuse to allow the termination of pregnancies that endanger the mother's life, dallying over how far a pregnant person's health must deteriorate before an abortion is no longer a mortal sin but instead a lifesaving procedure. Those who approve such terminations are often at the mercy of church officials, who not only review the case, but also decide if the medical practitioner involved has earned excommunication from the church based on his or her actions.

The issue came to a head in 2009, when an Arizona nun approved a lifesaving abortion in a Catholic hospital for a mother of three who was eleven weeks pregnant. The hospital medical board ruled that due to the woman's pulmonary hypertension, continuing the pregnancy would likely have killed her, and recommended an abortion before the fetus developed further and placed additional stress on the woman's heart. Because of this decision, Sister Margaret McBride was reassigned from serving on the ethics committee of St. Joseph's Hospital in Phoenix, as well as excommunicated from the Catholic Church. "I am gravely concerned by the fact that an abortion was performed several months ago in a Catholic hospital in this diocese," Bishop Thomas J. Olmsted told the *Arizona Republic*. "I am further concerned by the hospital's statement that the termination of a human life was necessary to treat the mother's underlying medical condition. An unborn child is not a disease. While medical professionals should certainly try to save a pregnant mother's life, the means by which they do it can never be by directly killing her unborn child. The end does not justify the means."[1] Bishop Olmsted eventually revoked St. Joseph's status as a "Catholic" institution when doctors at the hospital refused to agree not to provide an abortion if the same situation presented itself again. The hospital refused to capitulate to the Bishop's demands, saying, "Morally, ethically, and legally we simply cannot stand by and let someone die whose life we might be able to save."[2]

Bishop Olmsted, like many of the faith who work with religious institutions and their associated health care entities, believe that it is always better to err on the side of faith rather than on the side of women's health, and that adhering to the tenants of faith outweigh the right of the patient to receive needed care. "[T]he equal dignity of mother and her baby were not both upheld," Olmsted said at a news conference. "The mother had a disease that needed to be treated. But instead of treating the disease, St. Joseph's medical staff and ethics committee decided that the healthy, 11-week-old baby should be directly killed."[3] However, the only "treatment" available to save the woman's life was to end her pregnancy—there was no surgery, medication or other option that could successfully treat her condition. The incident became just the most public of the many complaints that the American Civil Liberties Union had sent to the government informing them of Catholic health institutions that have denied women care due to "moral objections." "No woman should have to worry that she will not receive the care she needs based on the affiliation of the nearest hospital," said Brigitte Amiri of the ACLU Reproductive Freedom Project, in a July 2010 report on the state of emergency reproductive care in religiously-affiliated hospitals.[4]

As more hospitals merge, the dominance of religiously-affiliated hospitals has only grown more pronounced. According to the Catholic Health Association of the United States, as of January 2019, more than one in every seven patients is cared for in a Catholic hospital, and adding in other denominations brings that number up to one in six.[5] As a result of these mergers, more emergency rooms, surgery centers, maternity wards and ICUs are under rules that demand that medical care be "consistent with church teaching." In rural areas where there is often only a religiously-affiliated hospital option, this means that more pregnant people than ever are finding that their care is a secondary concern, with an existing or future pregnancy being the hospital's top priority.

It is this strict devotion to faith over medicine that makes the spreading refusal of services under the guise of "conscience" such a threat to reproductive health. And with a federal judiciary that has dramatically shifted rightward on religious exercise freedom claims—especially now that the benches are being stacked by the Trump administration—the conscience-based political movement benefits from broad legal cover. We already saw the groundwork being laid during the Obama years in cases like *McCullen v. Coakley*, where the Supreme Court struck down a Massachusetts buffer zone ordinance at abortion clinics as being unnecessarily large and infringing on the religious liberty and free speech rights of protesters, or in the birth control benefit case of *Burwell v. Hobby Lobby*, where the Court extended the scope of the Religious Freedom Restoration Act to some privately-held nonprofit businesses, ruling they could file a religious objection to complying with the benefit and object to their employees having access to insurance plans that covered abortion and contraception, granting evangelicals a new legal opening to launch conscience objections to *other* laws such as state non-discrimination statutes.

Resolution of future cases involving "religious liberty" will likely depend on those precedents, and build off Supreme Court victories that have upheld the constitutionality of a host of statutes found to be "particularly burdensome" to women, including twenty-four hour waiting periods and the ability to use Medicaid to pay for an abortion. As a result, there is every reason to believe that the Court will find conscience clause legislation, or challenges to reproductive health care requirements based on individual beliefs, acceptable due to the fact that they create similar burdens in the form of "increased costs and potential delays."[6] In the meantime, religious conservatives continue to push for additional concessions related to contraception and abortion—and discrimination regarding GLBTQ rights as well—while arguing to the public that individual religious freedom is under assault by government overreach.[7]

Religious objections to providing reproductive health care or access to such care is an issue in state courts as well. The Supreme Courts of New Jersey and Alaska both found their state conscience clauses unconstitutional as applied to nonsectarian hospitals because the clauses infringed upon constitutionally protected reproductive rights. In those cases, the state courts required private, nonsectarian hospitals to provide abortion services, even though those services conflicted with the hospital's religious beliefs.[8]

•

Sam Brownback has long been familiar with the debate over faith trumping medicine. As a U.S. senator, Brownback was as radically opposed to abortion, contraception and family planning as any politician in Congress.

He received a perfect rating from the National Right To Life Committee in 2006, and a rating of zero from NARAL Pro-Choice America in 2003.[9] Brownback also fought to have the Fourteenth Amendment cover the "preborn" and for the government to legislate that life began at the moment of conception, as well as opposing funding to reduce teen pregnancy with contraception and fact-based sex education.[10] He became even more devoted to anti-women's health policies once he was elected governor of Kansas in 2010.

Despite the fact that Dr. George Tiller, known for providing abortions into the third trimester, had a clinic in the state, Kansas has never been known for its liberal stance on reproductive choice. Quite the opposite, as the state has long been the literal center of the anti-abortion movement, with groups like Operation Rescue moving to Kansas for the sole purpose of putting pressure on Tiller to shut down his practice. During Democratic Kathleen Sebelius' time as governor from 2003 to 2009, anti-abortion activists tried to create as many legal roadblocks to obtaining abortions in the state as they could, although most of those restrictions were vetoed by Sebelius. But after she was appointed Health and Human Services Secretary by President Barack Obama in 2009, the only thing standing between the extreme anti-abortion Kansas legislature and the decimation of women's reproductive rights in the state was gone. "Kansas provides a perfect example of two kinds of Catholics," explained Meghan Smith of Catholics for Choice, a progressive reproductive health policy organization. "We had Governor Sebelius, who was a pro-choice Catholic, and while she was governor talked about being a pro-choice Catholic, and we immediately had Governor Sam Brownback, who was an anti-choice Catholic. Both of them are Catholics, and both of them talk about their faith, and both of them approach this issue from two very different places."[11]

The Brownback era ushered in an immediate focus on limiting abortion in any way possible. Brownback signed bills restricting abortion access and removing coverage of abortion from state—as well as private—insurance plans. He also sought to eliminate family planning money from Planned Parenthood and to close down the state's few remaining abortion clinics by passing legislation that would force the clinics to spend tens of thousands of dollars in upgrades or else be shuttered (These "Targeted Regulation of Abortion Providers" or TRAP laws will be discussed in more detail later). Still, that wasn't enough, as the governor soon received a set of bills that would create the most expansive protections yet for those who refused to provide medical services on the grounds of "conscience."

Kansas, like many other states, already had a bill on the books that protected individuals being asked to participate in an abortion by allowing them to refuse. Despite this, religious leaders and their followers began to push the definition of "participation" to extreme forms, and in the process established precedents that continue to this day. For example, in 2010, a bus driver in Texas argued that he was illegally terminated from his position after he refused to drive a woman to a Planned Parenthood clinic, believing that the woman was about to undergo an abortion. Edwin Graning, an "ordained Christian minister" who was defended by former evangelical leader Pat Robertson's American Center for Law & Justice, received a $21,000 settlement from the Capital Area Rural Transportation System, which chose to pay Graning rather than fight the suit, which they believed would cost even more to defend.[12] Graning actually never knew for sure that the woman he was driving was going to have an abortion, but said that he had his wife call the clinic and that the recording said if a woman is having complications, she should go to the hospital. "I'm a Christian . . . I love the Lord and I'm not going to be a part of something like this," Graning told *LifesiteNews*. "I pastored years ago, and I've done a lot of things—and normally I wouldn't have made any issue out of this—but you know, I'm really getting tired of Christians getting kicked around. I mean, we see other things as going on in this country, and somebody somewhere along the line is just got to quit bending the knee to Baal and letting this government run over us."[13]

Edwin Graning wasn't the only one to take the definition of assisting in an abortion to an extreme. In 2011, a group of nurses in New Jersey sued their employer for being "forced" to participate in abortions at the University of Medicine and Dentistry of New Jersey. Their definition of participating, however, consisted of checking women into the hospital, taking vital information like blood pressure and temperature, entering the patient's name into a computer and walking them out of the center after the abortion was over. The lawyer for the nurses defined assisting in an abortion to be anything, no matter how tangential, that involved a patient seeking an elective abortion procedure. "If they did that, they'd be helping to make it happen," Attorney Demetrios Stratis told the *Star-Ledger*. "They're doing much more than that, obviously."[14]

At least the New Jersey nurses who objected to participating in an abortion weren't putting anyone's life in danger. In 2010, a pharmacist at a Walgreens store in Idaho invoked the state's "Freedom of Conscience for Health Care Professionals" law and refused to fill a woman's prescription for the drug Methergine, which is meant to control bleeding, saying that she believed it was likely being used in abortion aftercare. Kristen Glundberg-Prossor of Planned Parenthood of the Great Northwest, told the *Boise Weekly*, "We have heard of a lot of accounts where individuals across Idaho are being refused, but this is the first incident that we know of involving one of our own nurse practitioners. [Methergine] is neither an abortifacient or contraceptive. But the pharmacist asked our practitioner, 'Do you need this because of an abortion?' Our practitioner told the pharmacist in keeping with federal law, she couldn't disclose that. And then the pharmacist said she wouldn't fill the prescription. When our practitioner asked to speak to another pharmacist, she was hung up on."[15] Although Walgreens reprimanded the pharmacist for not passing the prescription to a colleague to be filled, the Idaho Board of Pharmacy refused to take any action on the complaint, arguing that the state's conscience clause was "not under board domain."[16]

Jon O'Brien, the president of Catholics for Choice, says that cases like these are attempts "to prevent someone else from trying to exercise their freedom of conscience." According to O'Brien, if "what you do impedes on someone else's free exercise of will, I don't believe that is a conscience situation. That is impeding someone else from being able to do what they need to do. I think that is wrong ethically and morally. I can tell you it's wrong as a Catholic, but I can also tell you it's wrong from the point of view of respecting other people and being honest in the way we do things."[17]

The state of Kansas, however, believed that "conscience" was open to limitless interpretation. In early 2012, two bills proposed in the state legislature sought in different ways to allow for greater designation of what fell under moral objections to "assisting abortions" as well as expanding what was considered a "taxpayer-funded" abortion. H.B. 2598, the "No Taxpayer Funding for Abortions" Act, went beyond the scope of the Hyde Amendment, which prohibits the use of Medicaid funding for any abortions except in cases or rape, incest or the health of the pregnant person, by seeking to eliminate the University of Kansas Medical Center's program to train doctors on how to perform abortions. The bill stated that since the center was funded with taxpayer dollars, providing abortion training was tantamount to paying for abortions. Previously, students who wanted to learn abortion care as part of their schooling (common surgical abortion procedures are used in miscarriage management as well, making them a regular part of any OB-GYN training) left campus and went to a Planned Parenthood clinic to be trained. H.B. 2598 sought to end that practice.

H.B. 2598 also defined any entity that was associated with the state's public schools to be taxpayer-funded, meaning that no employee, contractor, or even school volunteer could be associated with an abortion provider. In an attempt to ensure that members of Planned Parenthood or similar groups would not be allowed to inform students about health issues or offer age appropriate sex education, the bill would ban members of those organizations from volunteering at schools, even if their tasks were unrelated to health education. And, in one of the most unusual aspects of the bill, the state proposed what amounted to a sales tax on abortion of 6.5 percent tax on every medical exam and procedure associated with the actual termination. On top of that, H.B. 2598 would also end tax credits for companies that did any kind of business with abortion providers, as a disincentive to forming any sort of financial relationship. Elizabeth Nash, state issues manager for the Guttmacher Institute, told *Raw Story*, "This is a complete turnaround in this idea of small government. Somebody spent hours, if not days, combing through the entire Kansas tax code to find every spot where you could possibly prevent abortion providers from being a non-profit healthcare provider. It's really amazing. The bill is 68 pages long. Somebody spent days trying to figure out how to manipulate the tax code to disqualify abortion providers. That is a level above and beyond what we have ever seen."[18]

Introduced during the same legislative session as H.B. 2598, H.B. 2523 made the unprecedented move of proposing that conscience clauses shouldn't just cover drugs that actually caused abortions (i.e. RU-486), but should also "bar anyone from being required to prescribe or administer a drug they 'reasonably believe' might result in the termination of a pregnancy."[19] When writing legislation, language like "reasonably believe" and "might" are loaded and intentionally vague terms that leave those in charge of administering medication or filling prescriptions with enormous power. Although the Kansas state legislature said that the language was meant to apply only to filling medication abortion prescriptions (something that almost never occurs in a pharmacy due to the highly restricted distribution of RU-486 by its parent company), doctors and reproductive rights advocates noted that by adding the word "might" the legislature opened an avenue for pharmacists to refuse to fill birth control pills and emergency contraception as well, such as the so-called "morning-after pill." "When the bill went to committee it was clear from the testimony that was given by the pro-life side that the bill was about contraception," said Holly Weatherford, Program Director of the ACLU of Kansas and Western Missouri, adding that:

> They had pharmacists testify that they believed contraception was abortion and they didn't want to then administer or fill prescriptions for birth control. When the bill actually went to the floor in front of the full chamber in the House, the author of the bill described it simply as dealing with abortion and sterilization and unfortunately the legislators didn't know the law well enough to understand that Kansas has had longstanding conscious refusals in law in Kansas for abortion and sterilization. We did hear in some of the comments on the House floor that some of those pro-life legislators knew exactly what the bill was about and they made off-the-cuff comments about needing to protect against people having mail-order abortions, referring to emergency contraception, but in the end it passed overwhelmingly.[20]

Despite medical evidence to the contrary, the Food and Drug Administration's official literature on the "morning-after pill" (also known as "Plan B") states that one possible way the medication works is to inhibit the implantation of a fertilized egg in the uterine lining.[21] In 2012, the *New York Times*, after doing its own scientific research and contacting medical experts, declared that the FDA's statement simply wasn't true. "The notion that morning-after pills prevent eggs from implanting stems from the Food and Drug Administration's decision during the drug-approval process to mention that possibility on the label—despite lack of scientific proof, scientists say, and objections by the manufacturer of Plan B, the pill on the market the longest," reported the paper. "Leading scientists say studies since then provide strong evidence that Plan B does not prevent implantation, and no proof that a newer type of pill, Ella, does."[22]

Updating FDA labeling is a grueling, expensive and often highly political task, as we saw with the decade-long effort to update the protocols around RU-486, and one that the companies producing emergency contraception drugs saw little reason to undergo, considering so few people likely to use the medication would be discouraged from doing so because of the mistaken impression it could stop a fertilized egg from implanting. However, that refusal emboldened anti-abortion activists, who still insist on calling emergency contraception, as well as the birth control pill itself, an abortifacient. For those who believe that a fertilized egg is the equivalent of a living breathing person, use of emergency contraception is considered an abortion. For the rest of the medical profession, however, which understands that a pregnancy cannot begin until after implantation (ask any person who has undergone in vitro fertilization if they are pregnant simply because they have fertilized eggs waiting to be implanted), it is understood that no pregnancy truly exists before implantation, especially since prior to that point a pregnancy test would remain negative.

Still, a very vocal batch of anti-abortion doctors, pharmacists and others continue to claim that contraception causes abortions, spurred on by groups like Physicians for Life and Pharmacists for Life. As a result, a growing number of medical practitioners are refusing to prescribe contraception, citing their own religious beliefs. Dr. Gabrielle Goodrick, a family planning and abortion practitioner in Arizona, noted the rising number of doctors who are refusing to prescribe contraception to their patients, citing their own religious beliefs. She told the story of one doctor who decided that for Lent, she'd stop offered tubal ligations, or even birth control itself. "A drug rep came and told me this and I didn't believe it and she said, 'No, it's absolutely true. This is what she told her staff and they had to cancel patients and patients that wanted birth control had to see someone else.' I don't think it's malpractice," Goodrick continued, "I think they can do that. But I've had patients come in here with unplanned pregnancies. They had gone in and seen their doctor for their annual and said 'Okay I need my birth control' and the doctors said 'Oh, I'm sorry, I don't prescribe birth control,' and they're like 'What am I supposed to do?' and the doctor says 'You'll have to schedule with another provider.' They won't even get another doctor to write them the prescription and so then they end up here."[23]

Jon O'Brien of Catholics for Choice believes that the consciences of individuals should be respected, but "if you are a pharmacist or a doctor, and even if you are against contraception, it doesn't mean within Catholicism that you have to refuse it to someone else. You can be a Catholic pharmacist, you'll never use contraception, it's against my religion, but you still could prescribe it and be a good Catholic. That's the way my religion actually works." O'Brien also says that the health of the patient should never suffer because of the conscience issues of the provider. "But let's say you are a Catholic doctor and you don't want to perform the abortion or fit the IUD, or you don't want to prescribe the pill. I say okay. As a woman, I wouldn't want them performing any sort of procedure on me that they feel uncomfortable doing. So it's partly about protection of the patient or client. But the most important thing is that the end user should not have to suffer as a result of your conscience."

In addition to increasing the number of drugs covered under a conscience clause, H.B. 2523 would have also expanded the definition of who could be considered a "provider." Although the language in the bill was assumed to refer to medical professionals such as doctors, nurses, health care providers and pharmacists, there was no guarantee that it couldn't be extended to anyone who happened to be in charge of handing out medication. As an example, in Florida, a rape victim was denied access to the second of two pills comprising a dose of emergency contraception when a prison guard refused to provide it to her, citing moral objections. The victim, who had an outstanding warrant for failure to appear in court, was arrested and jailed when she showed up at the police station to report that she had been raped. She had already been examined and given the first dose of medication at a health clinic, but the second pill, which was confiscated when she was put in jail, was kept from her by the whim of the guard in charge.[24]

•

Both H.B. 2598 and H.B. 2523 were heatedly debated in the Kansas legislature, then substituted into senate bills that had already passed committee. However, H.B 2598 died in the senate, based mainly on a fear that the University of Kansas Medical Center could lose accreditation if it did not allow students to learn how to perform abortions, which are considered a basic component of gynecological care.

Unlike its counterpart, however, H.B. 2523 passed through the Kansas senate, and was signed into law by Brownback on May 14, 2012. The bill was designed to facilitate conscious refusals for contraception, but as the ACLU's Holly Weatherford explains:

> There is a common misunderstanding of the ban, which is 'What's the big deal if someone doesn't want to prescribe birth control or emergency contraception, they shouldn't have to.' But their follow-up is always that they should then refer patients to where they can receive those services. This bill includes a referral ban which means that hospitals and organizations don't have to require physicians to refer for certain services. Kansas is a managed-care Medicaid system. That means women need referrals for services to be provided so the referral ban is simply another barrier for women.

These barriers particularly harm those in the western part of the state. "These are a low-income rural population that might have one pharmacist within a thirty-mile radius, which is a significant distance for someone to travel who might not have the means to travel," Weatherford explained. "And then you're also looking at affordable health care, so a lot of people will use a Planned Parenthood or a federally qualified health center, and there might not be one for four or five counties. As we see more and more restrictions to women's health being passed and implemented in Kansas I believe we are also seeing a shift from focusing on targeting providers to targeting the patient, targeting women."

As if that were not enough, pregnant people in Kansas had another worry when accessing reproductive care: Operation Rescue getting a hold of their names and addresses. In the spring of 2012, the anti-abortion organization made the stunning announcement that it was in possession of the records of at least eighty-six women and girls who had been treated in one month at an abortion clinic in Kansas.[25] Just exactly how Operation Rescue came into possession of this information remains a mystery. Clinic officials confirmed a break-in around the time Operation Rescue claims it came into possession of the records, but the clinic didn't have reason to think any patient data had been breached. Regardless of how it came into possession of the information, Operation Rescue's plan was to turn the records over to the state and file a complaint against the provider. In the meantime, it posted the records online after the group went through each file to redact the patient names and other identifying information.

Cheryl Sullenger, Operation Rescue's senior policy adviser, said that a confidential informant had provided the papers and that no laws had been broken in their acquisition. "It's no secret we seek information about abortion clinics," Sullenger said. She wouldn't explain how the group got the records, essentially offering up "trust us" as evidence no laws had been broken. The Brownback administration then initiated an investigation against the clinic based on Operation Rescue's allegations that providers failed to report cases where a pregnancy was the result of incest or involved a minor to state health authorities. The clinic denied the allegations and challenged the group in court.[26]

In the end, bills like H.B. 2598 and H.B. 2523, as well as the actions of groups like Operation Rescue, revealed the strategy that was unfolding in the state of Kansas: Regulate abortion out of existence, and whatever can't be regulated out of existence will be terrorized into submission. That strategy is being replicated all across the country today as clinics close, protesters and other anti-abortion activists get more aggressive in their tactics, and the Trump administration extends "religious liberty" rights through executive orders and by setting up a new "religious liberty" office within the Department of Justice to ensure that no one's religious beliefs are being trampled by federal law (with religious beliefs primarily defined as those found in the Christian bible).

As the Supreme Court solidifies its conservative majority, and as Republicans continue to pack the lower courts with judges committed to overturning *Roe v. Wade*, we can no longer expect the judicial branch to save us from the overreach of the religious right as they tear down the barriers between church and state. In fact, with the assistance of the administrative and judicial appointments of the current administration, religious beliefs are now powerfully weaponized, with a conscience clause the most powerful trump card of them all.

11

ARIZONA

UNDERMINING THE
DOCTOR/PATIENT RELATIONSHIP

When Republican Jan Brewer replaced Democrat Janet Napolitano as governor in 2009, the residents of Arizona were quick to learn exactly how vital a gubernatorial veto could be when it came to protecting reproductive rights. Brewer, the former Arizona secretary of state, took over when Napolitano was selected by President Barack Obama to be the new secretary of homeland security. The move may have improved the safety of Americans across the country, but Arizona residents were left vulnerable to a state legislature determined to undermine the right to safe, legal abortion, birth control, and other reproductive services.

Following Brewer's ascension to the governor's office, emboldened by the knowledge that pretty much any bill they passed would automatically receive her signature, conservative politicians in the Arizona legislature went to work on an anti-abortion omnibus bill which "essentially revamp[ed] abortion policy in the state."[1] HB 2564 added a twenty-four hour waiting period after mandatory counseling from a doctor prior to an abortion, extended the ability for providers to invoke a conscience clause, and added restrictions for teens trying to obtain an abortion.

That was only the beginning. In 2011, the state passed HB 2443, the first Prenatal Non-Discrimination Act (PRENDA), a "race and gender based" abortion ban which made it a felony if a doctor was proven to have performed an abortion on a person who chose to terminate a pregnancy because of the race or gender of the fetus. While the ban itself was more conjecture than anything else—after all, how exactly would one be able to know the motive of a pregnant person terminating a pregnancy unless the patient told the provider in the first place—the idea behind the ban was to make providers nervous about potential liabilities for abortions they performed, as well as create an additional hurdle between patients of color and abortion providers. "That's one piece of legislation that really affects immigrant women because it kind of creates racial profiling of women," said Veronica Bayetti Flores of the Center for Advancing Innovative Policy. "Obviously legislation like PRENDA really targets immigrant women because it puts a lot of fears at the hand of the provider and the patients and again targets women of color, particularly immigrants."[2]

In addition to PRENDA, the state also passed HB 2416 in 2011, which restricted who was allowed to provide RU-486, as well as banning telemed. This two-pronged approach left some clinics in the state unable to perform abortions. Planned Parenthood—Arizona challenged HB 2416 as significantly increasing hardship for those who wanted access to legal first trimester abortions. "What we're specifically contesting are aspects of the legislation about nurse practitioners and physicians assistants providing this care, even though they have been providing this care in Arizona for over a decade with exemplary quality and safety ratings," Bryan Howard, president and CEO of Planned Parenthood Arizona, told *The Arizona Republic.* "There is no medical evidence that they should be prohibited from providing the care. And we know that given the shortage of physicians willing to provide this care, it will have a significant impact and place a burden on patients."[3]

While the rest of the country was watching the US Senate debate the Blunt Amendment in early 2012, a bill that would allow religious employers to refuse to add birth control or other medical coverage they found "objectionable" to their employee insurance plans, Arizona was about to go step further. The state senate approved HB 2625, which would allow employers to decide whether birth control pills should be part of an insurance plan based on what the employee in question was using them for. If it was for a "legitimate" medical condition, it would be covered. However, if a person was taking the pills to prevent pregnancy, then they would not be.

Beyond the potential violation of privacy involved in requiring workers to tell their supervisors about health conditions in order to obtain affordable medication, there was the added humiliation of patients being forced to provide medical proof that they weren't lying in order to obtain the pill. The sponsors essentially wrote the law saying that not only should a person not be given permission to control when they wanted to have children, they also couldn't be trusted to tell the truth about their physical health, either. The "she'll lie to get what she wants" argument isn't a new one, especially when it comes to pregnancy, as anti-abortion legislators have asked that rape and incest exceptions be eliminated from abortion bans based on the assumption that women would start lying about being raped just to get an abortion. In 2012, Idaho Senator Chuck Winder noted during closing speeches on behalf of the state's mandatory ultrasound bill in that, "I would hope that when a woman goes in to a physician with a rape issue, that physician will indeed ask her about perhaps her marriage, was this pregnancy caused by normal relations in a marriage or was it truly caused by a rape."[4] Winder later clarified that he meant that a woman would want to check and see if she was impregnated by her husband or by the rapist based on the age of the embryo or fetus, not that he necessarily thought they were lying about being raped. By that point, however, his words had been splashed across the national media, and the backlash was believed to be part of what forced the bill to be pulled.

More recently, abortion opponents have addressed this issue by requiring that exceptions on the grounds of pregnancy after a sexual assault require a police report made shortly after the incident occurred. The requirement serves two purposes. First, it harms those who are unwilling to report their assaults immediately (or at all), especially victims of date or acquaintance rape, which many on the right downplay as an actual assault, since they believe it isn't a "violent" attack by a stranger, but more a sexual encounter gone awry. Secondly, an assault survivor who reports a crime within a short window is more likely to receive emergency contraception at the time of the attack, making pregnancy less likely and eliminating the need for a "rape exception" (at least in cases where the use of emergency contraception isn't blocked as an "abortifacient.")

•

Also in 2012, the state of Arizona advanced SB 1359, a "Wrongful Birth" bill that would shield doctors from any sort of malpractice suit that developed as the result of the missed diagnosis of a fetal anomaly, especially one that might cause a woman to consider terminating her pregnancy. Sponsored by Republican Senator Nancy Barto, the intent of the bill was to eliminate the idea that "if a child is born with a disability, someone is to blame."[5] The passage of the bill would protect a doctor if they chose not to inform a patient that the developing fetus had a condition that could significantly impact its life.

That a doctor's judgment could trump the views of a pregnant patient when it came to that patient's own reproductive desires was already a practice among the most extreme of anti-abortion doctors, who often withhold medical information from their patients in order to ensure they didn't seek out an abortion due to a problem with the pregnancy. Dr. Gabrielle Goodrick of the Phoenix-based Camelback Family Planning, said that although it wasn't commonplace, it definitely happened. "I had a patient come in who was told she couldn't have an assessment of the pregnancy by ultrasound until twenty weeks," recalled Goodrick. "[Then] they are told they have to wait another four weeks for an evaluation or more detailed ultrasound to look for abnormalities. I think that it's already happening; a lot of the doctors here are extreme in their opinions. There are really conservative doctors here and they already aren't being forthright with their patients."[6]

If a doctor withholds relevant information in the course of diagnosis and/or treatment, and a patient relies on that incomplete information to give their informed consent, and they are later injured as a result, the doctor has committed an act of medical malpractice.[7] By withholding information to drive a particular medical outcome, the standard of care in "wrongful birth" laws would be set by legislators, not doctors. In practice, this meant that instead of an objective inquiry into the medical treatment and advice given to a pregnant person based on what the medical profession as a whole considered competent care, treatment would be determined by the individual beliefs of the doctor. This shifts the patient from the primary focus to, at best, a secondary consideration. If *Casey* tilted the balance to favor potential fetal life over actual maternal life, then wrongful birth bills break the scale all together, as those in states with these types of laws can never be sure the medical information they are receiving is accurate and unbiased, nor can they sue in the event that the information is found to be wrong or negligent. This requires pregnant patients in wrongful birth states to exercise greater caution and be even stronger advocates for their own care, as what constitutes accepted medical practice will no longer be easily determinable. Pregnant people would, in effect, have the same legal standing as juveniles or persons under legal guardianship and conservatorship, devoid of the ability to consent to a full course of medical treatment on their own.

Ultimately, the impact of these bills goes beyond abortion politics. For example, birth injury suits represent a significant portion of medical malpractice cases, in large part because the costs associated with an act of negligence in pregnancy and delivery are so great. Insurance companies typically (and usually successfully) fight coverage for those costs, meaning that malpractice recoveries often represent the only financial means for many families of providing for a disabled child. Wrongful birth bills will allow these claims to go uncompensated, because all health care professionals will need to do to avoid liability is to justify their course of treatment in terms of seeking to prevent an abortion. The creation of a medical malpractice shield strips women of the ability to be compensated for sub-standard medical care rendered to them while pregnant.[8]

Wrongful birth laws also completely shatter the trust necessary between a doctor and patient. How can a patient go through a pregnancy not knowing if they should believe a doctor who says the baby is healthy? Many patients may not even realize the position their doctor's views on abortion until they find themselves in a situation that involves a medically futile pregnancy. They are then often shocked by the news. Dr. Goodrick told the story of one patient who was warned that if anything was wrong with the fetus, she would still be expected to give birth. "Before the patient even said anything the doctor came in and said, 'If you have any testing or even if it's Downs, every baby deserves a chance at life.' The patient hadn't even opened her mouth and the doctor was already telling her the rules, that she would not support her if anything was wrong with the baby because every baby deserves life."

.

The reason it was so important for Arizona to make sure that doctors would be shielded from potential lawsuits if a baby was born with a previously undiagnosed disability that would normally have led a family to consider abortion was because the state was about to introduce HB 2036. The "Women's Health and Safety Act," would take the "fetal pain" abortion ban that Nebraska had passed in 2010 and twist it into a bill that would entirely change how pregnant people prepared for and dealt with potential complications in wanted, but medically flawed, pregnancies.

Although "fetal pain" abortion bans had been spreading across the country since Nebraska passed theirs in 2010, they had all been based on the same cutoff point—twenty weeks post fertilization, or twenty-two weeks gestation, a standard medical concept for dating pregnancies based on the woman's last menstrual cycle. With HB 2036, Arizona decided instead to set the cutoff for obtaining an abortion at twenty weeks gestation. By choosing to begin their ban two week earlier—based on the argument that "abortion becomes increasingly more dangerous than childbirth by twenty weeks gestation, with ever-increasing risk beyond twenty weeks"—not only would Arizona be further eroding the rights established in *Roe v. Wade*, but the state would be taking away a pregnant person's right to decide whether or not to carry to term a fetus that was genetically compromised or that faced major health risks.[9]

Most genetic issues or anomalies cannot be detected via ultrasound until close to twenty weeks gestation, which is why an anatomy scan isn't offered until that time in pregnancy. By creating a ban that would go into effect near or even before many patients would be likely to learn about such problems, the Arizona legislature was taking the decision about how to deal with such pregnancies out of the mothers' hands. Pregnant women would have to decide immediately whether or not to terminate their pregnancy, or be forced to carry doomed fetuses simply because they waited too long. A state that believed that a pregnant person should have to wait at least twenty-four hours after meeting with a doctor to terminate a pregnancy they didn't want now thought that pregnant people should rush into terminating a wanted pregnancy, possibly before having any sort of follow up and confirmation of any health abnormalities, simply to beat an arbitrary deadline.

These were the concerns that Dr. Paul A. Isaacson, an OB-GYN who works with high risk pregnancies, expressed when he testified against the bill in March 2012:

> In normal prenatal care, an ultrasound to assess the fetus is done in the 18–20 week range LMP. Prior to that range, an accurate fetal survey can't be done due to the small fetal size and immaturity of the organs. If an initial fetal ultrasound assessment shows a suspected abnormality, the patient is typically referred to a perinatolgy practice for a more thorough ultrasound. It might take several days for that to be arranged . . . If a severe fatal anomaly is confirmed, the woman may then need time to reach a decision about whether to terminate the pregnancy... For such women, this bill would force them to carry to term, often at substantial health risks to themselves.[10]

The legislature rejected Dr. Isaacson's plea, and in April 2012 passed HB 2036, which Governor Brewer signed. The law was scheduled to go into effect on August 2, 2012.

Unlike the Nebraska fetal pain bill, HB 2036 was challenged in court. On July 13, 2012, the Center for Reproductive Rights and the American Civil Liberties Union filed suit on behalf of Isaacson and two other Arizona physicians who claimed that the twenty-week gestational ban would harm their ability to meet the medical needs of their patients. "This law in Arizona displays a callous disregard for the complicated and very difficult circumstances many pregnant women face—and yet proponents of the law have the audacity to claim that it is designed to protect women," Nancy Northup, President and CEO of the Center for Reproductive Rights (CRR) said in a press release. The organization's lawyer, Janet Crepps, decried it as legislators playing doctor: "When state legislatures attempt to practice medicine, they get it wrong and women pay the price. By imposing criminal penalties, coupled with extremely narrow health exceptions, this law requires physicians to endanger the lives and health of their patients."[11]

Judge James Teilborg, an appointee of President Bill Clinton, presided over the hearing in US District Court for the District of Arizona. CRR's Janet Crepps presented a straight-forward challenge to the Arizona law, arguing that states are forbidden from banning abortions prior to viability. Teilborg disagreed, and asked Crepps a series of questions about which abortion procedures might be involved and the relative frequency of each. He then lectured Crepps for what he believed was a lack of compassion for the unborn, echoing the increasing concern in the federal judiciary over fetal rights. He said he had read the plaintiffs' affidavits and had found that they "reflect profound compassion and concern for their patients, the women, and presumably the fathers." However, he added, "I didn't find anywhere in those affidavits any expression of concern by the plaintiffs' positions for the unborn child—or even a hint of concern on their part." That was when it became clear that Teilborg was ready to take on *Roe*. "Given that silence on that part," he continued, "and given the silence in your own presentation, doesn't that underscore the legitimacy of the state's regulatory action out of concern for the unborn child?"[12]

On July 30, 2012, Teilborg issued his order and refused to block the law from going into effect. Pending emergency intervention, Arizona had just successfully enacted the most restrictive abortion bill in the country at the time. Perhaps more importantly, Teilborg's decision set up a question that seemed perfect for the Supreme Court to grab onto: in light of the *Gonzales* decision banning partial birth abortions both pre and post viability, what other pre-viability bans can survive constitutional scrutiny? For Teilborg, HB 2036 was constitutional because it wasn't a ban, but a regulation. "HB 2036 does not prohibit all abortions after 20 weeks gestational age. Rather, HB 2036 regulates abortions that take place after 20 weeks gestational age" wrote the judge. "Accordingly, HB 2036 does not purport to ban all abortions past 20 weeks gestational age. Further, the statute allows for abortions up to and including 20 weeks gestational age. As such, HB 2036 is not a ban on previability abortions, but is rather a limit on some previability abortions between 20 weeks gestational age and viability (which usually occurs between 23 and 24 weeks gestational age)."[13]

Once Teilborg did away with the idea that viability posed any true obstacle to finding HB 2036 constitutional, he attacked the Plaintiffs' arguments that the ban would force pregnant people to carry to term fatally flawed pregnancies because most fetal anomalies are detected outside the twenty-week window:

> Plaintiffs argue that a pregnant woman needs time to make the extremely difficult decision as to whether to continue the pregnancy and, in such a situation, it will take longer than twenty weeks to make such a decision. Accepting these statements as

true, while HB 2036 will make it necessary to make an immediate decision as to whether or not to have an abortion in some cases, such a time limitation cannot be construed to be a substantial obstacle to the right to make the abortion decision itself.[14]

One of the footholds justifying Teilborg's decision was the fact that that HB 2036 arguably impacted only a small pool of potential victims in the state—those seeking abortions between twenty weeks and twenty-three weeks.[15] While the number of people potentially injured by a law shouldn't matter—a law should be no less constitutional because it injures the rights of a few—a 2006 Supreme Court decision found that anti-abortion bills that only restrict the rights of a few pregnant people are not unconstitutional.[16] In *Ayotte v. Planned Parenthood of Northern New England*, the Court refused to strike down a New Hampshire parental notice law because it would only affect a small number of people. The law prohibited doctors from performing an abortion on a minor until forty-eight hours after written notice was provided to her parent or guardian. The law included a judicial bypass provision (allowing the minor to seek a court order permitting the abortion without her parent's knowledge) and an exception where an emergency abortion was needed to prevent the minor's death. Before the law took effect, three abortion clinics and an abortion doctor filed suit seeking to overturn it on the grounds that in a small percentage of cases, a minor's health would be threatened without a "prompt abortion." The state of New Hampshire asserted that the judicial bypass provision would allow for a prompt abortion in such cases.

The Supreme Court ruled that striking down the law on its face was not necessary or justified since only a few applications of the law would present a constitutional problem. The opinion in the case was drafted by Justice Sandra Day O'Connor. It would be the last of her career before she retired from the court, and the decision seemed to reflect this fact, as the opinion goes out of its way to find a reason to support the law, or as much of it as possible. "When confronting a constitutional flaw in a statute," she wrote, "we try to limit the solution to the problem. We prefer, for example, to enjoin only the unconstitutional applications of a statute while leaving other applications in force . . . to sever its problematic portions while leaving the remainder intact."[17] Legislatures were now essentially free to pass laws they knew were in direct conflict with *Roe*, with the promise that those laws would be allowed to go into effect while constitutional challenges played out. Furthermore, the opinion made clear, those future challenges would have to come from individual women or providers who had suffered an actual injury and could challenge the law "as applied" to them. By clearly favoring "as applied" challenges to abortion laws, the Court had erected yet another barrier for those needing abortion care. If *Gonzales* had provided anti-abortion legislators the roadmap to follow in providing sufficient evidence to make sure their abortion restrictions survived constitutional review, then *Ayotte* was an example for courts in upholding abortion restrictions that were drafted specifically in conflict with established precedent.

•

The Center for Reproductive Rights filed an immediate appeal of Judge Teilborg's decision. The Ninth Circuit Court of Appeals then issued an immediate emergency injunction blocking HB 2036 from taking effect while the constitutionality of the law was appealed.[18] Both legislators and attorneys for the state of Arizona were eager to use HB 2036 as a direct legal challenge to *Roe*, hoping the Ninth Circuit would give them exactly the outcome they hoped for, and one that at that point previous "fetal pain" bans failed to provide.[19] Should abortion opponents receive a favorable opinion allowing "fetal pain" to be a new standard for creating abortion bans, they could then introduce more medically disproven "science" claiming a fetus could feel pain earlier and earlier, until abortion would be impossible to access before the gestational limit was reached.[20] As a result, pregnant people who lived in states that don't affirmatively legislate to protect reproductive health would find themselves with no access at all. Without a change in course, it would no longer matter what *Roe* said: those who could become pregnant would be legislated and adjudicated out of full and complete citizenship.

But once again, abortion opponents failed to get the ruling they so desperately wanted. In May 2013, the Ninth Circuit Court of Appeals upheld the injunction that blocked Arizona's ban from being enforced, saying the state "may not deprive a woman of the choice to terminate her pregnancy at any point prior to viability." Arizona responded by appealing to the Supreme Court, but in January of 2014 the body rejected the opportunity to revisit or overturn the lower court's ruling, settling the matter for HB 2036.

Unable to advance the ball on the twenty-week ban strategy, Arizona returned to the more successful task of undermining the doctor/patient relationship between pregnant patients and their providers. In March 2015, Republican Representative Kelly Townsend added an amendment to SB 1318, a bill seeking to keep abortion coverage from being allowed in insurance plans introduced in the state's insurance exchange. The amendment mandated that physicians who terminated pregnancies using medication abortion state that there were ways to "reverse" the procedure, using a new and at that point completely unproven technique known as "medication abortion reversal." The theory behind medication abortion reversal was that if a pregnant patient took mifepristone, but didn't take misoprostol as a follow-up, they could "reverse" the effects of the initial pill by taking large amounts of the hormone progesterone. But there were a number of reasons why this theory couldn't be proven in medical circles. In order to conduct clinical trials, a group of patients must act as a placebo group in order to prove that the treatment is more effective than no treatment. That's obviously not an option for people undergoing the "reversal" in order to remain pregnant. Plus, patients are only offered the progesterone treatment if there is still an embryonic heart tone or fetal heartbeat before the progesterone is given. As a result, it was impossible to know if these patients were truly having successful reversals because of the therapy, or simply having failed medication abortions in the first place, with progesterone having absolutely no effect positively or negatively in keeping the pregnancy sustained. "If [a patient] is having thoughts of not taking the second pill, I don't give her the first pill," Dr. Goodrick told *Rewire News* when the amendment was introduced.[21] "It is just insulting to her intelligence to imply that she isn't capable of making a decision and following through with that decision. We trust women can make their decisions as consenting adults."

Despite the unreliable nature of the data provided by "abortion reversal" supporters and no study of the potential long-term effects on a pregnant person or the eventual pregnancy, Arizona lawmakers decided that "abortion reversal" as an option should be immediately added to the state's informed consent information provided prior to an abortion. Much like the assertion that abortion causes breast cancer, depression and premature birth, abortion providers in the state would also be required to tell the patient a medication abortion could be reversed and offer a website for patients to contact for assistance if they change their minds. The bill and the amendment passed but was blocked by a federal lawsuit soon after. Republican Governor Doug Ducey repealed the bill in 2016 rather than continue litigating the case.

•

Despite the failure of SB 1318, Arizona found yet another way to pit abortion providers and patients against each other, this time over the idea of fetuses somehow managing to "survive" an abortion attempt. In 2017, legislators passed SB 1367, which required doctors to make sure that "all available means and medical skills are used to promote, preserve and maintain the life" of any fetus "delivered alive," regardless of the likely long-term health outcomes of that fetus.[22] The bill requires abortion clinics to have neonatal emergency equipment and staff trained on neo-natal resuscitation if they perform abortions after twenty weeks, in the unlikely event of a live birth. Traditionally, for fetuses after about twenty weeks gestation, clinics doing second trimester care will inject digoxin into the heart of the fetus to assure that there is no potential for a mistaken live birth—as well as to be positive they don't accidentally fall in danger of either the 2002 Federal Born Alive Act or the 2007 Partial Birth Abortion Ban. Despite the protocol, SB 1367 added mandates meant to saddle clinics with additional costs or make them consider dropping how far in gestation they will offer terminations—or maybe close down altogether.

The new mandates are complicated, expensive, and, of course, completely medically unnecessary. There are no instances after the protocol went into effect of fetuses "surviving" an abortion, or any transfers to hospitals to prove that the new ordinances are solving any sort of lapse in care. This didn't stop extreme Republicans from pushing for a similar law at a national level, however, as the same requirements were written into Nebraska Senator Ben Sasse's "Born-Alive Abortion Survivors Protection Act," which failed to pass in early 2019.[23]

"Born Alive" bills are one of the most vicious ways of pitting doctor and pregnant patient against each other by using the criminal code as leverage. For a doctor providing a later abortion—because of a fetal anomaly, a medical issue in the pregnancy, etc.—the pregnant patient should be their first responsibility. If somehow the fetus manages to make it through an abortion (a scenario that is purely fictional), the state would then step in to redirect the doctor's care, placing the fetus as the new priority even if it wasn't viable due to gestational age or other medical concerns. Not prioritizing the fetus puts the doctor in danger of a jail sentence, loss of medical license or other punishment, and forces that practitioner to violate the wishes of the pregnant person—his first and true patient.

Of course, the likelihood of such a scenario occurring at all is extremely slim, but the real goal of such legislation—to sow mistrust between a doctor and the pregnant patient—is very real. And it is unsurprising that it first came from Arizona, where the trust factor when it comes to reproductive health has long been dangling by a thread.

12

MISSISSIPPI

CLOSE THE CLINIC, BRING BACK THE COAT HANGER

A patient walking through the doors of the Jackson Women's Health Organization clinic in Jackson, Mississippi needs to be prepared. As the only provider of abortions in the entire state, the clinic is rarely without at least one protester lying in wait for any women who may be entering with the intent of terminating a pregnancy. A patient may run into Dana Chisholm, currently vice president of Pro-Life Mississippi, who will sing hymns, quote Bible tracts and offer to pray with her, or one of the "fresh air" fire and brimstone preachers of Operation Save America and Abolish Human.[1] (Fortunately, patients no longer have to worry about Roy McMillan, an elderly anti-abortion activist who passed away in 2016 and took a more aggressive approach by yelling "Mommy, please don't kill me mommy! I have a dream, mommy!")

Jackson Women's Health Organization has been the sole public provider of abortions in the state of Mississippi since 2004. As such, the clinic has become a lightening rod of controversy in a state that very much disapproves of pregnancy termination. This controversy reached a head on Election Day 2011, when Amendment 26, declaring support for "personhood"—which defines life as beginning at the moment of conception, as well as granting legal rights to the fertilized egg—appeared on the ballot. The personhood movement had already failed in Colorado, where a similar ballot initiative had been voted down twice. But Mississippi, with its devout Christian population and staunchly anti-abortion leanings, was considered the ideal state for finally getting a foothold into redefining a person as the moment sperm and egg meet.

Amendment 26 became the hottest topic in the 2011 state election—even more heated than the race for governor. (Perhaps one of the reasons the governor's race was less controversial was that both the Republican and Democratic candidates came out in favor of Amendment 26.)

Despite the intense groundwork of Personhood USA, a group that believes persons are "'created in the image of God' from the beginning of their biological development, without exceptions," Amendment 26 was solidly defeated, with 58 percent of the voters declaring they did not believe legal rights should be granted at the moment of conception.[2] A vigilant public relations campaign that kept voters informed about the legal ramifications of the amendment—that it could make some forms of contraception, especially IUDs and possibly even the birth control pill, illegal, that infertility treatments could be outlawed, and that people who miscarried could potentially find themselves investigated by the authorities—cooled the public's interest in granting rights to fertilized eggs, even if it could end abortion in the state.

One of the leaders of the grassroots informational campaign was Jackson Women's Health Organization itself. Owner Diane Derzis formed "Wake Up Mississippi" as a vehicle to campaign against Amendment 26. In an open letter pleading for funds to help her new group, Derzis reiterated the need to defeat the amendment not just to keep abortion legal in Mississippi, but everywhere else as well:

Legislators and anti-choice zealots continue every year with their assaults on reproductive healthcare making MS abortion laws the most restrictive in the land. AND...We are still standing STRONG! However, on November 8th, the MS ballot will include the Personhood Amendment which will end abortion in MS and will more than likely take Roe v. Wade to the Supreme Court. WE CANNOT ALLOW THIS TO HAPPEN! And neither can you . . . If passed, Personhood Amendment #26 will not only ban abortion BUT ALSO ban most (if not all) forms of birth control, end in-vitro fertilization, and make stem cell research illegal. In addition, women who miscarry will be subject to criminal investigation! THIS MEASURE GOES TOO FAR AND IS A THREAT TO—NOT ONLY WOMEN IN MISSISSIPPI—BUT THE ENTIRE COUNTRY! [3]

The 2011 election also ushered Republican Phil Bryant into the Mississippi governor's office. A co-chair of the "Yes on 26" campaign, Bryant advocated for Amendment 26 so thoroughly that his staff passed out bumper stickers supporting the amendment during campaign events. Prior to election day, Bryant told *Salon* that the fight over Amendment 26 was "a battle of good or evil." "[T]he evil dark side that exists in this world is taking hold. And they're saying, what we want you to be able to do is continue to extinguish innocent life. You see, if we could do that, Satan wins."[4]

Nothing strikes at the heart of *Roe v. Wade* the way the concept of fetal personhood does. The entire premise of a constitutionally protected right to abortion pivots on a balance between the actual life of the pregnant person and the developing life of a fetus and assumes those two actors, living mother and developing child, are not always equal. Fetal personhood laws upend this balance, moving "life begins at conception" from an aspirational statement to one with legal consequences.

The first legal notions of personhood came in 1989, when the Supreme Court, in *Webster v. Reproductive Health Services*, considered a challenge to a Missouri anti-abortion law that, among other items, had in its preamble a statement that the life of each human being began at conception and that state law may be interpreted to give unborn children the same rights enjoyed by other persons. Writing for the majority, then Chief Justice William Rehnquist noted that the preamble did not regulate abortion, but merely expressed a judgment favoring childbirth over abortion, a judgment that prior case law, specifically, *Maher v. Roe*, permitted. But the Court added that if the state were to use the preamble to limit the conduct of the plaintiffs as abortion providers, this might present a justiciable issue at a later date. The Court further observed that the preamble had applications in other aspects of state law, such as tort and probate law, and to give it full-force-and-effect could expand it beyond the legislative intent. On whether or not a declaration that life begins at conception is constitutional, for the time being, the Court did not comment, since it did not present an issue ripe for review.

Justice Blackmun, joined by Justices Brennan and Marshall, led the dissenters. Blackmun accused the Court of attempting to erode *Roe* by endorsing, even tacitly, a legislative statement that directly conflicted with precedent and women's civil rights. Blackmun would have struck down the preamble because, in his view, it would chill the exercise of a right to an abortion and unconstitutionally burden the use of contraceptive devices. In a separate dissent, Justice John Paul Stevens wrote that the preamble violated the Establishment Clause because it adopted an essentially religious view. He also wrote that he believed it would impact contraceptive use in violation of the Court's precedent on that issue in *Griswold v. Connecticut* and similar cases.

The anti-abortion makeup of the court has only grown stronger since the *Webster* decision in 1989, with the addition of Justices Clarence Thomas, Samuel Alito and of course Chief Justice John Roberts. Now that conservatives Neil Gorsuch and Brett Kavanaugh are also on the bench, that's a five-person majority that likely supports the Missouri preamble in context at the very least, and possibly full-blown personhood for fertilized eggs as it relates to restricting abortion and contraception in a worst-case scenario. That anti-abortion advocates see in *Webster* and the right-ward shift in the court an opening to attack *Roe* is evidenced by ongoing efforts to push for personhood even in the face of crushing rejection by the citizens of the states proposing it. That legislative effort finally hit its ultimate goal in May of 2019, when the state of Alabama passed a full abortion ban from the moment of conception, with absolutely no exceptions for anything short of the life of the pregnant person being in immediate danger—a direct and blatant challenge to *Roe* (and the autonomy of any person who can get pregnant) itself. Simply put, there is an all-out war on reproductive rights underway under the guise of "personhood" that started in Missouri and is spreading across the nation. And in many ways, Mississippi was the front line of that war.

•

The defeat of Amendment 26 was just a temporary victory for pro-choice advocates in Mississippi, as multiple abortion bans were the proposed during the state's 2012 legislative session. Like in Ohio, Mississippi proposed a ban on abortion after the point in which an embryonic or fetal heartbeat could be detected. Although the bill passed the house, the senate chair of the judiciary committee refused to allow a vote, saying he had no interest in passing a law that was so obviously unconstitutional. However, unlike in Ohio, anti-abortion legislators in Mississippi tried to do an end run around the committee chair, as house leaders attached the ban as an amendment onto a separate bill that changed the maximum prison sentence for someone charged with child homicide. The bill once more passed the house, but stalled in the senate when the chairman again refused to let it out of committee for a full vote. The senate's refusal to pass either the heartbeat ban or a second ban not allowing RU-486 to be dispensed unless a doctor was present in the room caused abortion opponents to refer to the state senate as a "chamber of death." However, the senate won back the approval of anti-abortion activists when it passed HB 1390 in April 2012, a TRAP (Targeted Regulation of Abortion Providers) bill that they hoped would end elective abortion in the state of Mississippi once and for all.[5]

Traditionally, TRAP legislation is meant to enact backdoor abortion bans by restricting access to clinics via an incremental process that usually harms just a few providers at a time. A TRAP law will, for example, limit the locations of clinics in order to force providers into costly moves, or prohibit their ability to move to more accessible locations. The legislation may also limit who can provide abortions or do the pre-screening, in order to reduce the number of patients who can be seen. Some proposed TRAP bills have introduced expensive new insurance requirements in an attempt to make it too costly for doctors to continue to offer terminations. Other TRAP laws, such as one passed in Kansas, create onerous rules for buildings that house clinics, including requiring extra wide doors for gurneys, regulating the size of "operating rooms" and even supply closets, as well as requiring that additional drugs be kept on site and changing licensing requirements for those who dispense them, even if those drugs bear no relation to the procedure being performed. (Kansas even mandated blood pressure cuffs for infants and toddlers, despite the fact that there would never be a need for those to be used in clinics.)[6] The ultimate goal of TRAP laws is to drive up costs in the hopes that clinics will be forced to close, or that doctors will refuse to do terminations due to expensive coverage and liability (or else add the expenses to the cost of the procedure, making it unaffordable for most women).

Although they are often used to try to shut down clinics and make abortion more difficult to access, TRAP laws usually do not attempt to eliminate abortion access altogether. However, Mississippi chose to go straight for the knockout blow when it came to HB 1390. Like most pieces of TRAP legislation, the bill was based on the misguided idea that abortion is a risky, dangerous medical procedure, and that patients need to be protected and kept safe in case something goes wrong. The bill's proponents brushed away the evidence that, especially in the first trimester, abortion is actually much safer than childbirth, and that the risk of complications is extremely low. Instead, they framed terminating a pregnancy as an effort fraught with potential life-threatening side effects in order to mandate who should be allowed to perform the procedure, and under what circumstances.

HB 1390 proposed that only board certified OB-GYNs be allowed to perform abortions, and that those doctors must have admitting privileges to a nearby emergency room in case of a complication that required immediate attention. It was the second point of the law that left Jackson Women's Health Organization in a bind. While all three of its staff physicians were board certified, only one had admitting privileges to a local hospital, and getting privileges for the remaining two physicians was unlikely in a state so adamantly opposed to abortion. Because of threats and intimidation, most of the doctors at the clinic didn't reside in state, making it more difficult for them to get privileges from a local hospital. The only doctor associated who had admitting privileges, Carl Reddix, had been targeted for that relationship by the state's lieutenant governor. Despite the fact that Dr. Reddix had already been serving on the Mississippi Board of Health for nearly a year—and that he had been appointed to the position by pro-life Republican Haley Barber—Phil Bryant's predecessor, Lieutenant Governor Tate Reeves, informed Reddix that his affiliation with Jackson Women's Health Organization made him unqualified to continue to serve on the board of health. Upon blocking Dr. Reddix's confirmation to the board, a spokesperson for the lieutenant governor said that Reeves, "had concerns about the appointment because of [Reddix's] affiliation with the abortion clinic and wanted Gov. Bryant to refer a qualified doctor to guide state health policy."[7]

Were admitting privileges really necessary to protect a woman's health, as the legislators alleged? Not at all, according to Dr. Jen Gunter, an OB-GYN, writer, and women's health advocate:

In the small likelihood there is a complication of a procedure it is not necessary (or sometimes even desirable) that the doctor doing the surgery correct the problem. For example, I am a gynecologist. I cannot fix every single complication of the surgeries that I perform. If I inadvertently damage the bowel during a hysterectomy I need a general surgeon to help me. If we extended HB 1390 to all surgical procedures (and we really should if it is for safety purposes) then no surgeon could do any surgery of any kind because no surgeon is trained to fix every single complication. Why single out women getting abortions? Shouldn't every patient at a surgical center benefit from the same law?"[8]

Dr. Gunter's explanation shows how the very essence of a TRAP law is to target directly those who provide abortion, and only them.

Mississippi was not the first state to propose that doctors have admitting privileges if they performed abortions. Alabama, Arizona, Indiana, Kansas, Missouri, Oklahoma, South Carolina and Utah had similar requirements in place at the time, all of which withstood court challenges. However, in the case of these other states, the act of obtaining or not obtaining admitting privileges wasn't something that would cut off access to safe, legal abortion entirely. "If the intent of the bill and the result of the bill are to shut down the only provider in the state, it may raise different constitutional questions than were raised in other cases where admitting privileges were an issue," Jordan Goldberg, state advocacy counsel for the Center for Reproductive Rights, told the *Associated Press*.[9] That continued to remain the difference between HB 1390 and other states' TRAP laws.

Lawmakers in Mississippi were unabashed about their intent to close the Jackson Women's Health Organization and end access to legal abortion in the state. When questioned about what would happen if HB 1390 forced the only clinic in the state to close, Senate Public Health Committee Chairman Dean Kirby said "[t]hat's what we're trying to stop here, the coat-hanger abortions. The purpose of this bill is to stop back-room abortions."[10] Coat hangers seemed to be an obsession for abortion opponents in the Mississippi state legislature. State Representative Lester "Bubba" Carpenter told supporters at a GOP event that although HB 1390 could end up in court, in the meantime, it would hopefully have stopped abortion in the state. That is, unless a pregnant person had a coat hanger available. Caught on video, Carpenter said, "It's going to be challenged, of course, in the Supreme Court and all—but literally, we stopped abortion in the state of Mississippi, legally, without having to—*Roe v. Wade*. So we've done that. I was proud of it. The governor signed it into law. And of course, there you have the other side. They're like, 'Well, the poor pitiful women that can't afford to go out of state are just going to start doing them at home with a coat hanger. That's what we've learned over and over and over.' But hey, you have to have moral values. You have to start somewhere."[11]

Carpenter's comments were a refreshing bit of honesty from a legislature that for the most part continued to use the guise of "women's safety" as a means of banning abortion. However, Diane Derzis was unmoved by their alleged concern. "These people hide behind words like 'safety,' 'women's health,' 'concern' and 'compassion,'" she told *Politico*. "This kind of legislation—they bring [it] up every year. Up to this point we've jumped through the hoop."[12] This time, the hoop was just out of reach, as Governor Bryant eagerly signed the bill into law on April 16, 2012. "This legislation is an important step in strengthening abortion regulations and protecting the health and safety of women. As governor, I will continue to work to make Mississippi abortion-free," Bryant stated once the legislation had passed through both chambers. On the day he signed the bill, he was much more forthright. "If it closes that clinic, then so be it."[13]

Governor Bryant might have been trying to make Mississippi "abortion-free," but in reality, he and his legislative cohorts were only making it inaccessible for lower income pregnant people—especially pregnant people of color. In 2010, nearly 2300 abortions were performed in Mississippi, the vast majority at the Jackson Women's Health Organization clinic.[14] Most of these abortions were performed on those who were "nonwhite, unmarried, had a high-school degree or less and already had children" and who claimed a "lack of financial and personal stability" as reasons for choosing a termination.[15] Closing the clinic would leave these people with three options. First, they could travel out of state to obtain an abortion, increasing their costs, even though many patients who seek abortions are already struggling financially. Second, they could continue the pregnancy, either adding another child they couldn't afford, or putting the baby up for adoption in the hopes that someone else would be able to raise it. Finally, they could try to terminate the pregnancy themselves, just like in the dark days before abortion was legal.

Under normal circumstances, the Jackson Women's Health Organization clinic would have had several months from the passage of HB 1390 to come into compliance, but the lawmakers demanded more immediate enforcement, aiming for a July 1 start date. House Public Health Committee Chairman Sam Mims sent a letter to the state health officer, Dr. Mary Currier, requesting expedited action on the bill, stating that he was looking into avenues to ensure that the clinic would not be allowed any sort of grace period to come into compliance. The state representative told *Reuters* that he did not "want to give the facility 10 extra days to perform abortions" and was discussing with lawyers the legality of asking for immediate action against the clinic.[16]

Deciding not to wait to be officially shut down, Jackson Women's Health Organization and Dr. Willie Parker, an OB-GYN who traveled to Mississippi to do abortions at the clinic, filed a lawsuit demanding an injunction against HB 1390 going into effect. The suit, filed on June 27, 2012, requested that a federal judge block the legislation, calling it an unconstitutional attempt to eliminate abortion in the state of Mississippi.[17] Parker and the clinic were represented by the legal team at the Center for Reproductive Rights. "For years, we have been beating back Mississippi's underhanded tactics to close the only abortion clinic in the state," said Nancy Northup, president and CEO of the Center for Reproductive Rights. "Mississippi lawmakers' hostility to women and their reproductive rights does not give them license to violate their constitutional rights. This measure would force Mississippi women who are already facing difficult circumstances to travel hundreds of miles to a neighboring state to get an abortion. That is simply not an option for many poor and working-class women, and will certainly lead some to consider unsafe and illegal alternatives that pose grave risks to their health, lives, and reproductive future."[18]

A temporary restraining order was issued late on the evening of Sunday, July 1. The court met again on July 11 to discuss a permanent injunction, with the state arguing that the clinic could pose a safety hazard and that even if the law went into effect, it would take at least ten months for the clinic to be closed down completely. The Center for Reproductive Rights and Jackson Women's Health Organization argued that without the clinic, there would be no access to abortion within the state, a clear violation of undue burden under *Planned Parenthood v. Casey*.

Judge Daniel P. Jordan III, a Republican appointee, was stuck in an unenviable position. If he sided with the plaintiffs, he would set a precedent on what constituted undue burden. If he sided with the state, he would also set a precedent, in this case saying that a right to access a first trimester abortion was not jeopardized by there being no clinics in a state—a ruling that would allow the rest of the country to separate themselves into states where abortion was either legal or illegal simply by banning providers in their borders out of existence.

When Judge Jordan returned his decision late on a Friday evening, he showed that he had found a way to avoid both issues. He ruled that HB 1390 was legal, and that Mississippi could put the law into effect. However, he also ruled that the doctors at the Jackson Women's Health Organization would not face any criminal or civil penalties under the new law. "The Act will be allowed to take effect, but Plaintiffs will not be subject to the risk of criminal or civil penalties at this time or in the future for operating without the relevant privileges during the administrative process," stated Jordan. "This will maintain the status quo in this litigation because the Defendants will be precluded from taking action that they do not now contemplate while Plaintiffs will be permitted to operate lawfully while continuing their efforts to obtain privileges as they said they would."[19]

"The judge sort of punted on the substance for the time being," said Michelle Movahed, Staff Attorney at the Center for Reproductive Rights. "He really focused on whether he felt we had shown irreparable harm. Certainly, I think he signaled that he was not looking at it that way and our challenge is not confined to specific circumstances, the two doctors providing the bulk of the abortions at the clinic right now." The ruling actually did harm the clinic even as it remained free of criminal penalties for now, Movahed explained. "The clinic continues to try to find providers who can meet the needs of women in Mississippi and since they've been having to look for providers outside the state, a requirement like the admitting privileges requirement or the OBGYN requirement is going to artificially restrict the pool of providers they can draw from. By constricting the number of providers, that's going to have a serious impact on women's ability to access care."[20] In this outcome, Mississippi came to represent the starkest example of the floor-to-ceiling approach to challenging *Roe*. With only one provider in the entire state and a litany of restrictions on accessing abortion services, Mississippi lawmakers had nearly succeeded in making abortion legal-in-name-only.

What would it mean for Mississippians to live in a state that literally would offer no legal access to abortion? It would be devastating for a population that already struggles with one of the highest poverty—and child poverty and infant mortality—rates in the country. The Mississippi Department of Health contributes the loss of 10 deaths for every 1000 live births in the state to be due in part to the often unplanned nature of pregnancies, as well as a lack of quality prenatal care.[21] Jackson Women's Health Organization's Dr. Willie Parker saw this problem up close, growing up in the south and being raised in poverty, which is why he was fighting to keep the clinic open. "For me, being from the south, having been reared in poverty, and as an African American person in the south in particular, I began to feel a sense of responsibility. Mississippi has one of the highest poverty rates in the country. The poverty rate for Mississippi in general is 20 percent and it's 48 percent for African Americans. This is the context in which African American women are experiencing unplanned, unwanted pregnancies and it meant that, if that clinic closes, a large proportion of the women affected are black and poor. Having grown up black and poor in the south, that led me to conclude that I personally had a responsibility to do something about that."[22]

It's the cycle of poverty that the poor—which in Mississippi often also means the black population—find themselves unable to escape, particularly if they are not allowed to have control over whether or not they want to continue an unplanned pregnancy. "One of the ironies is the state of Mississippi has one of the lowest abortion rates in the country," said Parker. "The irony is it's an extremely low abortion rate, relatively speaking, and yet disproportionately it is made of women who are more likely to have one child or multiple kids. A woman who already has a child living in poverty, and we know that's much more likely to be an African American woman, the poverty rate is double for blacks versus whites in Mississippi. It's the perfect storm around why, if that clinic closes, disproportionately African American women are going to be affected."

If Mississippi already has one of the lowest abortion rates in the country, why has the state become such a target for anti-abortion politicians? It could have something to do with the state's legislative makeup. According to the *Mississippi Clarion Ledger*, Mississippi had the fifth lowest representation of women in its legislature, with women holding just 26 of 174 seats in 2011, just before the TRAP bill was introduced.[23] Pamela Merritt, reproductive justice activist from Missouri and co-founder of ReproAct, a reproductive justice direct action organization, says it is that lack of representation that makes it so easy for lawmakers to enforce legislative control over women's lives. "I think, as woman who works in politics and a woman of color, I don't see a lot of me. You don't see a lot of women. We are definitely not representative of what we are in the population and you certainly don't see a lot of women of color. What you really don't see working politics or lobbying politically are your average every day 'sista'. We are easy targets. The fact that we're not represented in government, we are challenged to speak truth to government, makes us an incredibly easy target."[24]

Without proper advocacy in government, the cycle of poverty that poor, rural and minority communities are already stuck in is further compounded when their reproductive rights are virtually eliminated by the cutting off of access to abortion. "Children are expensive and no matter what the right to life movement likes to say, children cost money and making money is hard," states Merritt. "For women who are not degreed and are probably not going to get a college degree, shift jobs become the norm. They tend to not have health insurance and they tend to not be very forgiving of needing to leave because your child has an ear infection. Every child that a woman has compounds that stress on her job and makes it less likely for her to stay in a work environment and move up the ladder. So there's that factor and I can't stress enough how the reality is that unhealthy people who have unplanned pregnancies have complicated pregnancies and complicated health outcomes. In a very unforgiving world it's very easy to wake up all of sudden and you are 30, you've got 3 children and you don't have choices, you have decisions to make and you have compromises to make and very often they don't allow for the kind of risk taking that people who are more affluent have."

•

Despite Judge Jordan's ruling that the Jackson Women's Health Organization wouldn't be penalized for failure to follow the new law requiring admitting privileges for doctors who performed abortions, the state of Mississippi nonetheless moved ahead with its efforts to shut down the clinic. Soon after the judge's order, the state made its initial inspection of the clinic to cite them for non-compliance with HB 1390. While there would be no fine for the doctors or the Jackson Women's Health Organization as a result, the inspection offered the state board of health the chance to start the clock on the ten-month process of shutting down the clinic for good. The year 2013 began with the state board of health informing the clinic that due to its non-compliance with the new law its license would be revoked.[25]

Twenty-thirteen also introduced a spreading plague of even more admitting privileges-based TRAP bills, including another one that also directly targeted the lone clinic in a state. On March 25, North Dakota legislators sent a bill requiring that the Red River Women's Clinic, the state's sole abortion provider, be required to close unless its doctor could get admitting privileges at a local hospital to perform any potential follow up necessary if there was a medical emergency. The problem? The only non-religious hospital the clinic could use had a strict policy of not offering admitting privileges unless the doctor could guarantee at least ten admissions per year. Red River Women's Clinic would never meet that criteria. "I've had one time that I've had to admit a patient in the last ten years," clinic director Tammi Kromenaker explained. "We are very selective about the physicians we hire for our clinic, because we know we are a target. As the only clinic in the state, of course we have worked to ensure that we have the highest quality doctors. I would never employ a doctor who had to admit ten patients a year. That would mean they were a terrible doctor."[26] Like Jackson Women's Health Organization, Red River

Women's Clinic sued the state in order to keep the law from closing its doors. The clinic also received an injunction, but the suit was put on hold in 2014 when Sanford Hospital agreed to break protocol and work with the clinic to get them the privileges they needed.

Since then, other states have eagerly stepped on the admitting privileges bandwagon, also hoping to close clinics within their borders. Wisconsin's admitting privileges law would have closed Affiliated Medical Services in Milwaukee, the state's only independent clinic and the only clinic doing abortions up to the legal state gestational limit. Alabama's would have closed three of the state's five clinics and limited abortion to just the first trimester of a pregnancy, but it was blocked by a federal judge in 2014, who said the state's history of hostility and violence at clinics made it too hard for doctors to find hospitals to partner with.[27] (Not blocked, however, was another portion of the same bill, which required multiple onerous, expensive and medically unnecessary building code changes to abortion clinics, which put two of those clinics out of business for months trying to meet the new requirements). Louisiana had its admitting privileges law blocked in 2019 once it was argued that the requirement would shut down all but one clinic in the state.[28]

In Ohio, however, the state took a slightly different track, and with a lot more success. The state's transfer agreement version of the TRAP law (requiring a clinic to have an agreement to transfer patients to a specific hospital, rather than the physician at the clinic having admitting privileges there) allowed the state board of health to tackle clinics one by one by addressing lack of partnerships with hospitals through the licensing board. By taking a clinic by clinic approach versus closing a large number at once, the state has been able to avoid the federal lawsuits that stopped TRAP bill enactment in Wisconsin, Alabama and elsewhere. Ohio's strategy paid off—by the spring of 2019, there were only seven full-service abortion clinics left in the state (two others provide just medication abortion), down from seventeen clinics in 2011. The state is also currently suing to close yet another clinic in Dayton.

•

Overall, if attempting to close abortion clinics by requiring admitting privileges generally ended up in a federal injunction, you would think that packaging those same admitting privileges into a new bill, and then adding more building code requirements—such as demanding that abortions only be performed in Ambulatory Surgical Centers, even if the procedure was medication only—would be quickly rejected as unconstitutional, too. But when the state of Texas decided to do exactly that in 2013, an extremely conservative Fifth Circuit Court of Appeals bit on the opportunity to uphold the restrictions, even as they closed almost all the clinics in that vast state. With SB5 abortion opponents finally achieved the goal that had been pushing for ever since the first twenty-week ban came out of Nebraska.

They had finally made it to the Supreme Court.

13

"THE BURDEN IS UNDUE"

WHOLE WOMAN'S HEALTH V. HELLERSTEDT
AND AN ABORTION RIGHTS VICTORY

When Texas State Senator Leticia Van De Putte entered the capitol floor on June 25, 2013, she knew she had to act quickly. The Democratic lawmaker from San Antonio saw a room in chaos around her. Despite her best efforts, Fort Worth Senator Wendy Davis's eleven-hour long filibuster had ground to a halt, and there was still several hours before the midnight deadline to vote on Texas Senate Bill (SB) 5. While Davis had held the floor for more than half a day, Republicans were now cleared to move forward with the final roll call vote.[1]

For Texas abortion opponents, it was surprising that Democrats had managed to put off the inevitable for as long as they had. SB 5, the omnibus abortion bill introduced by Republican State Senator Glenn Hegar, was a Frankenstein's monster of nearly every popular abortion restriction proposed by state legislatures across the United States over the previous two years—all of which had previously failed due to the Democrats' ability to block them from getting to the floor. The bill would make abortion illegal after twenty-weeks post-fertilization, based on the disputed idea of fetal pain at that point in pregnancy, and require all abortions to be done in clinics that met the same standards as ambulatory surgical centers (ASCs) even though most abortions are done via vacuum aspiration or medication and really aren't any sort of "surgery." For a medication abortion under the bill, a patient would be required to come to a clinic for a consultation, wait twenty-four hours, return to that clinic for mifepristone, then return after another twenty-four hours for misoprostol, then return yet again for a follow up two weeks later to be sure the abortion was complete. On top of all those requirements, no clinic could remain open unless the doctor performing an abortion also held admitting privileges at a local hospital—something that was nearly impossible to obtain in a highly conservative state like Texas.

Anti-abortion activists were confident that if passed, SB 5 would be the death knell for abortion access in Texas. By closing most of the clinics in the state through the mandating of unobtainable requirements, the few providers that remained open would be unable to assist all of the patients who needed care before it was too late for them to legally terminate a pregnancy. What abortion opponents had to do to make the bill pass the certain legal challenges was to claim that the regulations weren't about restricting care, but rather keeping patients "safe" by demanding clinics meet the absolute highest of medical standards—even if those standards were medically unnecessary.

Regardless of the major impacts that it would have on abortion access, SB 5 appeared to be in position to easily sail through to passage through a special session and be signed into law. Texas conservatives had ample power to push through their agenda, and that power had grown exponentially after the Tea Party election wave of 2010. Governor Rick Perry had made limiting abortion access a major part of his legacy, too, with actions like stripping Planned Parenthood from Texas family planning funding and pushing the state's mandatory ultrasound law as "emergency" legislation. Though all of the individual abortion bills had died during the regular session, Republicans had no doubt that the new package of restrictions would get through once all of the state's other business was out of the way, especially since the rules for getting to a floor vote were far more lax during a special session.

It was there that lawmakers got over-confident. Because the house version of SB 5 didn't originally contain the ASC requirement, there was a forty-eight hour wait between the house bill being amended and when the senate could vote on the final version. That left just one day in the session for debate and passage—leading to an ambitious plan by senate Democrats to see if they could run out the clock.

To try and make that happen, Senator Wendy Davis began to filibuster the bill, with no breaks for food, drink, using the restroom, sitting or leaning or allowing others to take the floor, or even straying too far off the topic of the bill itself. Republican senators, meanwhile, took turns watching Davis to see if she made any mistakes that would allow them to end her filibuster and call for a vote. In the Texas senate, it is three strikes (mistakes), and you're out.

For eleven hours, Davis spoke continuously, even reading letters from people who had received abortions and opposed SB 5 because it would severely restrict care. But at one point, when she brought up previous cuts to Planned Parenthood under another Texas bill, the GOP swooped in to object, calling the line of discussion "not germane" to SB 5. That was strike one. Her second strike came when a colleague helped her put on a back brace after hours of being on her feet. Republicans called it "assistance" and told her she had just one more try before she would be declared out of order and her filibuster finished for good.

With the clock inching closer to midnight and time running out, Texas

Republicans grasped for any excuse to call the third strike on Davis, however flimsy it may be. By this point the state capitol was filled with bodies watching the proceedings closely—and over 100,000 people watching a livestream of the event on computers all around the country. All of them were witnesses when, with just two hours left, the final point of order was called on Davis, as she was accused of once again going off the topic of the bill, this time by bringing up the state's 2011 mandatory ultrasound bill.

With Davis's filibuster dead, Texas Democrats worked diligently to continue to eat up the clock to reach their midnight goal. It was an effort that would have been impossible had it not been for Senator Leticia Van de Putte. Van de Putte had been absent from the chamber for most of the day while attending her father's funeral, and did not return until late that night when it began to appear as if Davis's efforts might fail. Like her fellow Democrats, Van de Putte was eager to delay the vote as long as possible, and assisted in getting the proceedings down to where there were just fifteen minutes until midnight. It was at that point that the presiding senator (a Republican) chose to ignore her, instead recognizing another senator's call for a final vote.

But Van de Putte wasn't done. "At what point must a female senator raise her hand or her voice to be recognized over the male colleagues in the room?" she demanded, to tumultuous applause and shouting.[2] That thunderous noise continued until after midnight, ending the special session without a final vote on SB 5.

Unfortunately, the Democrat's victory was short-lived, as Governor Rick Perry called another special session, and this time SB 5 (now known as House Bill (HB) 2) passed. Perry signed it into law on July 18, 2013.

While HB 2 was an omnibus abortion bill, not all parts of the law were challenged immediately in court. The restriction on abortion after twenty-two weeks gestation (twenty weeks after the last menstrual period) and new requirements that clinics follow outdated FDA protocols rather than medical best practices for medication abortion were both left to go into effect as state law. But the medically unnecessary building and doctor regulations were a completely different matter. HB 2 required that abortions only be performed in ambulatory surgical centers (ASCs) rather than ordinary clinics, even if those clinics were only doing vacuum aspirations and medication abortions and not more advanced procedures. Prior to the bill's passage, only abortions performed after sixteen weeks needed to be done in ASCs due to the slight increase in possible complications and the more involved process of a later gestation abortion. HB 2 also mandated that every doctor who performed an abortion have admitting privileges from a hospital fewer than thirty miles away.[3]

Together, these two restrictions created impassable hurdles for Texas clinics to navigate. Clinics that hadn't been offering later abortion care were looking at the choice of either moving to new buildings or undergoing major construction—either of which could cost millions of dollars. Even if they could afford the expenses, clinics could still be shuttered if they were unable to find a doctor with local privileges, or a hospital willing to offer privileges to doctors who already worked at the clinic. To prevent this, hospitals were quickly identified as the point of vulnerability for clinics, and pressure was put on them by anti-abortion activists to rescind privileges in order to cut off access for abortion care. In Dallas, for example, two doctors applied for and received privileges from University General Hospital when the admitting privileges rule went into effect on October 31, 2013. But the hospital revoked their privileges in March 2014, saying that allowing the doctors privileges was "disruptive" to the hospital and interfered with its "reputation." The doctors sued, accusing the hospital of discrimination against abortion providers, and the hospital eventually settled and reissued the privileges in June 2014.[4]

Despite the issues the two physicians had, it was still far easier for doctors to get privileges in large urban areas like Dallas than in more conservative and rural parts of the state. Within a few months of the admitting privileges rule being enforced, clinics were closing across the state, mostly in poor and rural areas. Whole Woman's Health closed two clinics—in Beaumont, Texas and in McAllen in the Rio Grande Valley—in March 2014. It was the McAllen clinic that was the greatest loss, leaving most of southern Texas with no provider at all. For communities along the border who were unable to go further into the state because of lack of documentation and immigration checkpoints, there was now no longer any access to a legal abortion. By September 2015, the state of Texas had only nineteen clinics remaining—less than half the number it had had prior to the passage of HB 2 two years earlier (and this was before the second part of HB 2—the new ASC building standards—had been put into place.)

This first wave of clinic closures caused a crisis in abortion access in Texas. Candice Russell, a Jewish Latina reproductive rights activist and abortion storyteller explained in 2016 how difficult she found it to obtain an abortion in the state, despite living in a city that still had open clinics, because there were so many people trying to access care. "Even though I lived in Dallas, where clinic closures had yet to happen, the influx of patients from all over the state meant that it was a two-and-a-half week wait to schedule the first of my two state-mandated appointments," she wrote of her experience for *Glamour*. "I worried what would happen if I couldn't make it to both appointments and how close to the 20-week ban cutoff I would be if I had to reschedule. Having to work through another three weeks of pregnancy was unbearable, but I had no sick days to rest. I thought about every single scenario that would prevent me from having the abortion I knew was right for me and I panicked."[5]

Rather than wait and worry, Russell took out a payday loan and flew to California, where she was able to stay with her ex-partner and get an abortion immediately. "No one should have to take out a loan to get a simple, five-minute healthcare procedure," she wrote, "and they shouldn't have to leave their hometowns for it either."

•

Experiences like Russell's were just one of the issues that drove providers to file suit against the two restrictions. Whole Woman's Health and the Center for Reproductive Rights (CRR) filed a challenge on April 2, 2014, with other Texas clinics joining with their own representatives. On August 29, 2014 US District Judge Lee Yeakel ruled in favor of the right to an abortion, stating that the additional ASC standards would create an undue burden on access and would be enjoined from going into effect. He also added that the admitting privileges issue that had closed down the McAllen clinic infringed on the constitutionally protected right to an abortion for those who lived in the Rio Grande Valley, allowing that clinic to begin operating again. "The court is firmly convinced that the State has placed unreasonable obstacles in the path of a woman's ability to obtain a previability abortion," Yeakel wrote.[6]

The victory was short-lived, however. Just five weeks later, on October 2, a three judge panel on the Fifth Circuit Court of Appeals overruled Yeakel and allowed the ASC standards to be enforced—a move that immediately shuttered twelve clinics in the state and left patients who had already begun their twenty-four hour waiting period without the option to legally have an abortion the next day, and administrators in limbo as to whether they would ever be able to open their clinics again.[7] "I was able to glean enough in five minutes to know that I was going to have to make that call that I was dreading, that I was going to have to call the clinics and tell them that they would have to cancel all of their patients," ACLU Attorney Brigitte Amiri—who represented two abortion clinics in Texas—told *Cosmopolitan* in 2014. "I called one clinic, the one whose cell phone number I had, and then I asked a colleague to call the other. I called the first one immediately. They were done seeing patients. So we talked about what we would need to do going forward, that they would have to close their doors. I told them we would just have to take it day by day in the court process . . . I don't know, if they have to close their doors, if they can just reopen months down the road if this decision is overturned. Obviously they have a staff that is like family to them, and they want those staff members to try to find other jobs in the meantime. They can't just hold on indefinitely and possibly reopen their doors when a decision comes later. They might not be able to do that."[8]

Fortunately, the restrictions didn't last long. On October 14, 2014, the Supreme Court stepped in and put the ASC standards back on hold, and allowed the McAllen clinic and a clinic in El Paso to reopen despite their providers not having admitting privileges, putting Texas back into the precarious landscape of abortion access . . . at least for a while.[9] Eight months later, on June 9, 2015, the Fifth Circuit ruled that the state could enforce all parts of HB 2 for all clinics except for Whole Woman's Health in McAllen, and even that clinic would be forced to follow more stringent staffing rules and could only serve a very localized community of patients.[10]

As for the mass of potential patients in West Texas that would no longer be able to access a clinic as of July 1, 2015 when the rules were again enforced? The Fifth District argued that they could simply cross the border into New Mexico for care—despite the fact that those clinics weren't subject to either of the regulations Texas had introduced in order to protect patient "safety."

The ten clinics affected by the ruling didn't end up closing this time, though, as legal representatives filed an emergency appeal to the Supreme Court, which blocked the regulations. On November 13, 2015, the Court agreed to take up the case of *Whole Woman's Health v. Hellerstedt* (John Hellerstedt was Commissioner of the Texas Department of State Health Services when the suit was filed). The US Supreme Court was now poised to hear its first case on abortion rights since *Gonzales v. Carhart* in 2006, and again test the "undue burden" standard from 1992's *Planned Parenthood v. Casey*. As both sides clearly realized, what happened next could change abortion rights law for decades.

•

Oral arguments for *Whole Woman's Health v. Hellerstedt* commenced on March 2, 2016. Thousands of protesters convened outside the courthouse on a sunny but crisp early spring day, while the line of people who had been camping out in hopes of gaining entry to oral arguments snaked around the block. Both Stephanie Toti, lead lawyer from the Center for Reproductive Rights, representing the clinics, and Texas Solicitor General Scott Keller, knew that their arguments would be geared toward wooing one justice in particular—Anthony Kennedy. Keller needed to convince Kennedy that the restrictions existed solely to protect the health of those seeking abortions, not to restrict their access and force them to remain pregnant. Toti, meanwhile, needed to make it clear that despite the Fifth Circuit's contentions, both sets of regulations provided no actual medical benefits and made it impossible for many pregnant people—especially those who were poor, undocumented, of communities of color and lived in rural areas—to access abortion.

When it came to abortion arguments, Kennedy was always going to be the deciding justice, but this time, his decision would have more impact than ever. Just one month before the start of oral arguments, Justice Antonin Scalia had passed away suddenly, leaving the Court down one judge. During the Court's decision to stay the Fifth Circuit's ruling and leave the twelve Texas clinics open while the case proceeded, Scalia was one of the four justices who sided with the Fifth Circuit and wanted the restrictions to go into immediate effect (the others were Chief Justice John Roberts and associate justices Samuel Alito and Clarence Thomas). Without Scalia, Keller knew he needed to bring Kennedy to the state's side if he wanted a split court and any chance of the law being upheld.

If the lawyers' arguments were clearly catered toward Kennedy, the questions and statements from the openly conservative and liberal justices on the bench were just as direct. Alito pushed Toti to prove that the restrictions from HB 2 were truly responsible for closing down the state's abortion clinics, saying, "Well, there is very little specific evidence in the record in this case with respect to why any particular clinic closed. Basically your argument is that the law took effect, and after that point, there was a decrease in the number of clinics." Justice Elena Kagan stepped in, noting that for the two weeks that the entirety of the bill was enforced, all but nine clinics closed. Once the stay was implemented and the ASC standards were removed, the clinics immediately reopened. "It's almost like the perfect controlled experiment as to the effect of the law, isn't it?" she asked. "It's like you put the law into effect, 12 clinics closed. You take the law out of effect, they reopen."[11]

Justice Ruth Bader Ginsburg also dismantled the state's "patient health" argument by demanding to know why Keller was including a clinic in Santa Theresa, New Mexico as one Texans could access if the El Paso, Texas clinic was closed by HB 2's "safety" regulations. "[I]f your argument is right, then New Mexico is not an available way out for Texas because Texas says that to protect our women, we need these things [admitting privileges and ASC standards]. But send them off to New Mexico where they don't get either—no admitting privileges, no ASC—that's alright," Ginsburg countered. "Well if it's alright for the women in the El Paso area, why isn't it alright for the rest of women in Texas?"[12]

That was a question that Keller simply couldn't address, and likely one of the many reasons that pushed Kennedy to side with Kagan, Ginsburg, Justice Sonia Sotomayor and Justice Stephen Breyer to strike down HB 2 on June 27—the final day of the Supreme Court's 2015-2016 term. The Court determined that both provisions placed "a substantial obstacle in the path of women seeking a previability abortion," and "constitute[d] an undue burden on abortion access."

The Court also added that, "when directly asked at oral argument whether Texas knew of a single instance in which the new requirement would have helped even one woman obtain better treatment, Texas admitted that there was no evidence in the record of such a case."

Justice Stephen Breyer authored the decision for the abortion-rights majority. Breyer is the Court's data nerd, a former law professor and administrative law expert with a reputation for offering up humorous, if rambling hypotheticals to attorneys during oral arguments. Breyer laid out, item by item, the number of places the Fifth Circuit got its review of the data wrong as to the effect of admitting privileges on the availability of reproductive care. The list went on for pages.[13]

The decision was not just important because it helped solidify the role of the federal courts in evaluating abortion restrictions. The question the Court was asked to answer in *Hellerstedt* was whether *Casey's* "substantial burden" analysis takes into account the extent to which laws that restrict access to abortion services actually serve the government's stated interest in promoting health?" For the first time since the 2007 *Gonzales* decision, the role of the judiciary in serving as a firewall for abortion rights was at issue. And the liberal wing of the Court, with Justice Anthony Kennedy tagging along, made it clear the courts had an important role still to play.

In upholding the Texas abortion restrictions, the Fifth Circuit Court of Appeals had relied heavily on a line of reasoning in *Gonzales* that said when there is a question of scientific or medical uncertainty, legislators could essentially pick a side they agreed with and draft laws accordingly. The Fifth Circuit extended that logic further in the fight over HB 2, ruling that once legislators announce their justification for an abortion restriction, there was little, if anything, the federal courts could do to second-guess that reasoning.

Not so, the Supreme Court ruled in *Hellerstedt*. "The statement [by the Fifth Circuit] that legislatures, and not courts, must resolve questions of medical uncertainty is also inconsistent with this Court's case law," Breyer wrote. "Instead, the Court, when determining the constitutionality of laws regulating abortion procedures, has placed considerable weight upon evidence and argument presented in judicial proceedings" holding that the *"Court retains an independent constitutional duty to review factual findings where constitutional rights are at stake."* Justice Breyer's opinion italicized that final clause for emphasis. The federal courts would not simply rubber-stamp legislation aimed at curbing abortion rights because lawmakers claimed the restriction would promote patient safety.

The five to three decision reopened many (but unfortunately not all) of Texas's clinics, and rippled out to other states as well. Alabama Attorney General Luther Strange immediately announced he would no longer be defending the state's own TRAP law that was at that point enjoined, but otherwise would have closed four of the state's five clinics. Wisconsin's legal battle to close their clinics died as well, as the Supreme Court refused to hear the state's challenge, calling it already settled. Within days of the ruling, Planned Parenthood Federation of America announced an ambitious plan to begin researching whether clinic restrictions in at least eight other states could now be challenged and removed.[14] "Undue burden" to accessing an abortion had finally been defined, and for the first time in decades, there was a genuine possibility that abortion access might finally be expanded.

That is, until the November 8, 2016, when everything completely changed yet again.

14

INTO THE TRUMP YEARS

AND THE BEGINNING OF THE END OF *ROE*

The Supreme Court decision in *Whole Woman's Health v. Hellerstedt* may have encouraged abortion rights activists eager to see restrictions finally being struck down at the highest level, but at the same time, it offered the right something they had been desperately searching for—a tool to unify their conservative base and motivate them to get to the polls that November.

Despite conservatives' common goal of ending legal abortion, the rise of Donald Trump in the Republican Party had fractured the base. By June 2016, it was clear that the real estate mogul and reality television star was going to be the next Republican nominee for president. While a handful of stalwarts dreamed of ways to block his nomination at the convention the following month, most of the political powers in the GOP were brainstorming how to get the highly religious evangelical wing of the party to show up and cast their ballots for a man with multiple ex-wives, a number of affairs, and no real religious convictions, whom many suspected might not be as opposed to abortion as he claimed on the campaign trail.

What was needed was a solid commitment from their new leader that he would allow the religious right full control of his administration if he won, and the best way to solidify that promise was in a contract with the anti-abortion movement. Enter the Susan B. Anthony List. On September 16, 2016, the anti-abortion organization—which earlier in the primary had been one of the biggest backers of the "anyone but Trump" campaign—announced that candidate Trump had committed to a full-scale pledge to the pro-life movement in the event that he won the White House. Susan B. Anthony List president Marjorie Dannenfelser was designated the national chairwoman of the presidential contender's Pro-Life Coalition, and according to a letter released by the group, a President Trump would make four commitments to the cause of ending abortion in the United States:

- "Nominating pro-life justices to the US Supreme Court.
- Signing into law the Pain-Capable Unborn Child Protection Act, which would end painful late-term abortions nationwide.
- Defunding Planned Parenthood as long as they continue to perform abortions and reallocating their funding to community health centers that provide comprehensive health care for women.
- Making the Hyde Amendment permanent law to protect taxpayers from having to pay for abortions."[1]

Of all his promises, it was the commitment to only nominating Supreme Court justices that would overturn *Roe* that pushed so many ambivalent Trump voters into showing up at the polls.

Due to the sudden death of conservative Justice Antonin Scalia in February 2016, and Republican Senate Majority Leader Mitch McConnell's refusal to hold hearings on President Obama's choice to fill Scalia's seat, the centrist DC Circuit Judge Merrick Garland, the Supreme Court had one open seat heading into the November 2016 election. Thus, the idea of only seating "pro-life" judges wasn't just a theoretical conceit, but one that far right voters saw as an immediate and consequential opportunity, coming at a time when it appeared that Scalia's death was about to solidify a solid pro-choice majority on the Court. With Scalia's seat still open, and the possibility of a Republican presidential win in November plus the likelihood of more Court vacancies to fill in the future, conservatives had the chance to alter the trajectory of the highest court in the nation for decades to come. If anything, the ruling in *Whole Woman's Health v. Hellerstedt* only made the need to control Scalia's seat even more urgent to anti-abortion activists.

It may not have been enough to win Donald Trump the popular vote, but the efforts paid off. According to a Pew Research Poll that analyzed the November 2016 results, 8 out of 10 white evangelical voters cast their ballots for Trump, an even larger pool of support than Mitt Romney in 2012, John McCain in 2008 or George W. Bush in 2004.[2]

If the religious right put their faith in Trump (or at the very least, the myriad of stalwart leaders who were backing him, ranging from Vice President Mike Pence to James Dobson of Focus on the Family, Family Research Council's Tony Perkins, Gary Bauer, the Copelands, Paula White, Jerry Falwell Jr. and more), they weren't disappointed. After his electoral college win, now President Donald Trump immediately filled his administration with social conservative activists and evangelicals, giving them prime cabinet appointments and roles in a variety of administrative departments—especially the Department of Health and Human Services (DHHS).

Abortion opponents filled the DHHS, bringing a completely new vision to a department that had been far more subtle about its political agenda under Democratic President Barack Obama. "The Trump administration stacked the HHS department with abortion opponents with records a mile deep and a decade wide," explains Mary Alice Carter, executive director of Equity Forward, a watchdog reproductive rights organization currently researching the Trump DHHS. "He's taken people from external special interest groups working against the policies at the HHS and now brought them in to undermine them from inside. It's everything from lawyers who worked to undermine the contraceptive mandate in the Affordable Care Act to people who supported abstinence only sex-ed."[3]

Most notably, the DHHS added language that supported the idea of "personhood" by defining life as beginning at the moment an egg is fertilized, codifying that into their mission statement in October 2017. "HHS is the US Government's principal agency for protecting the health of all Americans and providing essential human services, especially for those who are least able to help themselves," the revised Organizational Structure segment reads. "HHS accomplishes its mission through programs and initiatives that cover a wide spectrum of activities, serving and protecting Americans **at every stage of life, from conception** [emphasis added]. HHS is responsible for almost a quarter of all Federal outlays and administers more grant dollars than all other Federal agencies combined."[4] The obsession with potential embryonic and fetal life would come to guide a variety of DHHS policies, especially its stance on immigration and birth control.

The protection of potential fetal life came to a head in 2018, when Scott Lloyd was transferred from his role as the director of the Office of Refugee Resettlement (ORR). Lloyd had been at the center of the migration crisis, mishandling the family separations policy that allowed agents to steal young children and infants from the arms of parents entering the United States seeking asylum from their home countries, and throwing minors into camps while detaining and often deporting their parents, all without any attempts to reunite these families in the long run. These certainly weren't the acts of a department allegedly committed to public health—detaining children, separating them from their families and housing them in shelters with inadequate space, resources and medical care isn't exactly the healthiest environment for children. But it was Lloyd's repeated efforts to deny pregnant minors the opportunity to obtain an abortion that was the most remarkable example of the Trump administration's new "fetus first" agenda.

Lloyd's refusal to allow teens to access terminations came to the forefront in the case of "Jane Doe," a pregnant minor who sought a judicial bypass to avoid the parental notification law in Texas so she could end a pregnancy that was not discovered until she reached the United States. "Jane" was granted the bypass, but was blocked by the Office of Refugee Resettlement, which refused to allow her to leave her shelter in order to obtain the abortion.

"Jane" wasn't alone. According to memos uncovered by *VICE News*, Lloyd intervened in the abortion cases of several minors, either indirectly or directly attempting to coerce pregnant young refugees out of ending their pregnancies. The memos and depositions from the American Civil Liberties Union depicted an ongoing mission to keep teens pregnant against their will, forcing them to undergo counseling from anti-abortion "crisis pregnancy centers," and even in some cases, being counseled by Lloyd himself.

One teen even had Lloyd and his counterparts try to coerce her into undergoing the medically unproven "abortion reversal" procedure, which was discussed in chapter eleven. The teen, who was pregnant due to sexual assault, was taken to a hospital after taking her initial pill and forced into an ultrasound to see if a "reversal" was still possible. The ORR then sent an email to the clinic that provided the medication, asking if the proto-col for a "reversal" would work. Luckily the teen managed to take her fol-low-up medication within the recommended forty-eight hour window.[5]

Lloyd and his colleagues also suggested that while minor teens in detention did have the same right to an abortion that any pregnant teen citizen had, the government had the right to not "facilitate" the abortion in any way. It was that extreme definition of "facilitate" that allowed Lloyd and his cohorts to justify repeatedly blocking "Jane Doe" from an appoint-ment to terminate her pregnancy, hoping to deter her long enough that she reached the gestational limit for having an abortion, which is twenty weeks in Texas.

The gambit nearly succeeded, as it took over a month for "Jane Doe" to receive her abortion, after Lloyd and the ORR refused to grant her tem-porary release from custody to visit the clinic. "Jane" was eventually repre-sented by the American Civil Liberties Union, which sued the DHHS and demanded they give her access to her constitutionally promised procedure. On October 18, 2017, the ACLU obtained a court order to force Lloyd to release "Jane Doe" from custody to begin her abortion, and she was able to have the mandatory face to face pre-abortion counseling the following day. But the ORR then appealed the decision of the circuit court judge, prevent-ing "Jane" from having the actual procedure on October 20, as scheduled.[6]

The battle over "Jane Doe's" abortion made it to the US Court of Appeals for the D.C. Circuit, where the it was reversed and sent back to the same judge who had previously upheld Doe's right to terminate her pregnancy, who reiterated that opinion. While the Justice Department paused to consider whether to appeal to the Supreme Court, Doe's advo-cates rushed her to a clinic where she was able to immediately obtain a termination. She was already more than fifteen weeks pregnant.

Unfortunately, the case of "Jane Doe" wasn't an outlier, but a sign that the Trump administration would radically reinterpret the very definition of abortion rights. "We've seen an elevation of ideology over evidence in the HHS's interpretation of what the right to an abortion means when it comes to people in custody," says Equity Forward's Carter. "What we saw from Scott Lloyd at the Office of Refugee Resettlement was a fundamentally different reading of the right to access abortion in the United States for someone in the US." According to Carter, this new interpretation could eventually be applied to women in federal prisons, to public hospitals that get grant money from the government, and people being held in detention by Immigration and Customs Enforcement. "It was very disturbing to hear the government say where they believe the right to an abortion ends and where they can decide that for other people," Carter adds. "It was a very stark interpretation."

It was also a preview of the fight in the courts over abortion access that is currently unfolding. Trump's second Supreme Court appointment, Brett Kavanaugh, was a judge on the D.C. Circuit during the fight over "Jane Doe's" abortion, and issued an opinion that would have given the administration legal cover to run out the clock on her ability to access care. In response to losing the court battle and ultimately being unsuccessful in their attempts to block "Jane Doe's" abortion, the Trump administration, through its Solicitor General Noel Francisco, took the extremely unusual step of asking the Supreme Court to sanction Doe's ACLU attorneys for supposedly misleading the administration. Francisco, who had ties to the conservative litigation organization Alliance Defending Freedom prior to joining the Trump administration, cited no authority in his request, just the administration's outrage and contempt that they had been unable to prevent "Jane Doe" from obtaining an abortion. No career attorneys from the Department of Justice signed on to Francisco's claims, and the Supreme Court denied the request.[7]

In March 2018, following a lawsuit by the ACLU, a federal judge ruled that the Trump administration was not allowed to prevent pregnant, undocumented immigrant teenagers in custody from accessing abortion services. This ruling, at least temporarily, halted the administration's coercive policy blocking undocumented minors from obtaining terminations.[8]

•

At the same time that the Office of Refugee Resettlement was trying to force minors to remain pregnant (while ignoring conditions in detention camps that were leading to an increase in miscarriages among *all* pregnant migrants in their care), the DHHS was working to remove Planned Parenthood from its Title X family planning program. The department's aim was to replace the organization with centers that offered limited forms of reproductive healthcare services—primarily STI testing, pregnancy confirmations and abstinence-only education—but which did not offer any forms of hormonal or barrier method contraception.

Anti-abortion activists thought they had gotten a major boost in their "defund Planned Parenthood" campaign when President Trump was elected in 2016. By having Republican control of the House, Senate, and White House, abortion foes imagined that a bill defunding the organization would be within easy reach. But getting a defunding bill through Congress was much harder than it appeared on first glance. First, standalone legislative efforts would likely fail due to the Senate GOP not having a veto-proof majority. In addition, attempts to block funding by writing it into federal budget omnibus bills also wouldn't work. While President Trump may have been willing to shut down the entire government to obtain funding for a border wall between the United States and Mexico, he wasn't going to veto a budget just because it allowed federal tax dollars to go to Planned Parenthood.

It was here that the DHHS stepped in with a new plan. The department offered a revised rule that reinstituted a Reagan-era regulation that Title X funds could not go to any organization that performed—or even counseled or referred to—abortion services. This "gag rule" required that any group receiving funding must not only have a physical separation from an office that offered abortion, but a "financial" separation as well. "This rule finalizes requirements that ensure clear physical and financial separation between a Title X program and any activities that fall outside the program's scope," the new rule read. "This physical and financial separation will ensure compliance with the statutory requirement that Title X funding not support programs where abortion is a method of family planning—and is consistent with the plain text of Section 1008, legislative history, and case law . . . This rule will require Title X providers to maintain physical and financial separation from locations which provide abortion as a method of family planning."[9]

The assumption was that Planned Parenthood would find itself incapable of separating its abortion and non-abortion services to the rigid new standards set by the DHHS and would inevitably be forced to either stop providing terminations or take a major financial hit from which it might not be able to recover. As the Family Research Council's Tony Perkins explained in March 2018, "If President Trump reinstated Reagan's 'co-location' rule, Planned Parenthood could still get Title X funds, but they wouldn't be able to offer those services in the same clinics where they perform abortions. They'd have to split up their offices—probably at great expense. Ultimately, Planned Parenthood would be forced to choose between dropping their abortion services from any location that gets Title X dollars or moving those abortion operations offsite. Either way, it puts a major dent in the group's bottom line."[10]

A draft of the revised Title X rules overhaul was released in the *Federal Register* on June 1, 2018, and was subject to a sixty-day public comment period. This resulted in over 500,000 comments from doctors, lawyers and current and future patients of the program weighing in on the changes. Despite the fierce debate over the new rules, the finalized version published on March 4, 2019 met all of the criteria demanded by the religious right when it came to trying to remove Planned Parenthood from being a Title X grantee. The new rules also gave social conservatives something else to cheer about: the newfound ability to funnel federal dollars to their own anti-abortion advocates and organizations. While reproductive health clinics that offered or referred for abortion services were barred from receiving grant money under the new Title X rules, entities that opposed abortion were now welcome to apply for money through the system, in spite of the fact that they were not offering and had no future plans of offering hormonal or barrier-based forms of contraception.

In a sign of the changes ahead, in March 2019, the Trump administration announced a $5.1 million funding pledge over three years to Obria Group, a Catholic-backed pregnancy center franchise formerly known as Birth Choice before a name change in 2015. Run by CEO Kathleen Eaton Bravo, Obria said it expects to use the funds to expand its current work in California. "With this grant, the administration has opened up a new avenue of health care choices for low income and underserved women and their families in California," Bravo said in a press release. "Many women want the opportunity to visit a professional, comprehensive health care facility—not an abortion clinic—for their health care needs; today HHS gave women that choice."[11]

Obria may be able to serve the needs of those seeking a provider for STI testing or annual exams, but if those clients want to prevent pregnancies with the most reliable forms of contraception, they will have to go somewhere else. The group's website offers a section called "Birth Control Side Effects" which briefly skims through short summaries of methods like IUDs, the pill, the patch and condoms, focusing mostly on their adverse medical effects, before providing a paragraph of information on Natural Family Planning/Fertility Awareness. The section concludes by stating, "Please note, however, that Obria Medical Clinics does not prescribe birth control."[12]

Allowing religiously-backed organizations that don't support and offer all forms of contraception to become official grantees of a government program meant to assist low income and uninsured people with reproductive healthcare may appear to be an oxymoron, but it has become clear that putting the "family" back in family planning hasn't been President Trump's only gift to the religious right. In fact, his entire administration has been organized with the specific intention of widening the path for white Catholic and evangelical supporters to have their religious dogma elevated as official federal policy. Just four months into his presidency, Trump issued an Executive Order that allowed religious leaders to advocate for and campaign in favor of candidates and issues without fear of losing their tax-exempt status. Trump also gave additional support to religious institutions such as the Little Sisters of the Poor, which claimed that forcing them to comply with the Affordable Care Act by notifying the government of their religious objection to offering employees access to benefits plans with no co-pay birth control violated their faith.[13]

In January 2018, Trump expanded the Department of Health and Human Services role in protecting religious liberty as well, by forming a new "Conscience and Religious Freedom Division," which would provide DHHS with "the focus it needs to more vigorously and effectively enforce existing laws protecting the rights of conscience and religious freedom." The administration promised that the new division would "more vigorously enforce twenty-five existing statutory conscience protections for

Americans involved in HHS programs, in order to protect Americans who have religious or moral convictions related to certain health care services."[14]

The Department of Justice, led at the time by Attorney General Jeff Sessions, also jumped on the bandwagon with its own dedicated religious liberty focus, which in July 2018 evolved into a "religious liberty task force" that was empowered to protect religious groups from persecution. "Under this administration, the federal government is not just reacting— we are actively seeking, carefully, thoughtfully and lawfully, to accommodate people of faith. Religious Americans are no longer an afterthought," Sessions said in a speech announcing the new task force, adding that, "[T] his Department of Justice is going to court across America to defend the rights of people of faith."[15]

As a result of its change in focus under the Trump administration, the DHHS is now dedicated to ensuring that the "right to life" is upheld under all circumstances—from forcing teens to give birth against their will, to funneling money from comprehensive family planning organizations to faith-based, anti-birth control "medical" clinics. The DOJ, meanwhile, has switched its focus from protecting the civil rights of those in traditionally marginalized communities to ensuring the religious liberty of those who feel trampled on if they aren't allowed to enforce their own moral beliefs onto others in the public realm. Together, the two arms of government make a frightening team that could wreck devastation on the right to terminate—or even prevent—a pregnancy.

By 2019, the Department of Health and Human Services was just picking at the edges of what it could do to block abortion access. With control over the Food and Drug Administration (FDA), future actions could include any manner of new rules that could make it harder for a person to access emergency contraception or medication abortion; just reversing Obama-era policies such as allowing emergency contraception to be available over the counter and with no age restriction, or officially sanctioning the updated protocol for medication abortion that requires far less medication and fewer trips to see a doctor face to face, would make for big, backward-looking changes. The DHHS could also choose to withdraw the waiver it granted to Gynuity Health Projects to test out a full telemed abortion project in four US states, a program that could massively expand access to abortion by allowing medication to be mailed to patients once an ultrasound is performed by a local doctor and the pregnancy is confirmed and dated at less than ten weeks gestation.

Those who fear the impact of an extremely anti-abortion, religious right-led DHHS only need to look at the department's March 2019 move to close down AidAccess, a European-based medication abortion website run by Dr. Rebecca Gomperts of Women on Waves/Women on Web, an organization which seeks to bring accessible abortion to pregnant people in countries where the procedure is illegal. The site launched in April 2018, and quickly became the target of an FDA investigation. Because Gomperts was sending medication from overseas to areas in the United States where abortions were hard to obtain, the FDA sent a warning letter in March 2019 telling her to cease operations because she was facilitating the "introduction of a misbranded and unapproved new drug into interstate commerce." The FDA argued that because the pills the site offered weren't verified as the two brand name medications approved in the US, they could be potentially dangerous.[16] The real issue, of course, was political, as no patient had reported any adverse drug effects or made any complaint about the site. Gomperts suspended operations for two months, but then announced she would be resuming service in May 2019, in direct defiance of FDA orders.

While an anti-abortion, anti-birth control DHHS could put a stranglehold on any new progress in reproductive services—or roll those rights back a decade or more—the Department of Justice could ulti-mately be even more dangerous to abortion access. It is the DOJ that decides how to pursue those who harass, terrorize or even physically harm abortion providers, abortion patients, and clinic volunteers. And with the department now pledged to protect and uphold the reli-gious liberty rights of Americans above any other constitutional right, there is very real reason to be concerned that clinic harassment will be taken seriously, or that the FACE Act will be enforced by the Trump administration.

The FACE—or Freedom of Access to Clinic Entrances—Act was signed into law by Democratic President Bill Clinton in 1994 as a means of ending the ongoing harassment and violence outside of abortion clin-ics, and even in some cases at the homes of abortion providers. As the "res-cue" movement grew in power during the 1980s, activists escalated their actions from pickets and sit-ins to clinic blockades and invasions, in some cases shutting down clinics for days, with hundreds of people gathered in front of clinic doors, refusing to move until police physically dragged them away. The 1991 "Summer of Mercy" in Wichita, Kansas, brought in thou-sands of protesters, resulting in six weeks of coordinated activities meant to keep the city's three abortion clinics closed for as long as possible. While abortions were still being performed periodically throughout that time, full care for patients was sporadic and fraught with extreme waits and other hurdles, while police officers conducted over 2500 arrests (in some cases arresting protesters multiple times) in order to keep the clinics open.

While no other protest was nearly as successful as the one in Wichita, "rescuers" began to engage in increasingly aggressive clinic closure attempts. Many traded numbers for immobility—while fewer people were blocking entrances, those engaged in such activities were now using handcuffs, bicycle locks and even chaining themselves to junk cars and other immovable objects to extend the amount of time it took to have them removed. Other tactics included super gluing door locks, using butyric acid, even arson at clinics across the country.[17] Efforts also moved beyond the clinics themselves, with protesters picketing the homes of abortion providers, or swarming doctors' cars or otherwise cutting them off from going inside the clinics. The escalation continued unabated until 1993, when Dr. David Gunn was assassinated in Pensacola, Florida outside the clinic where he provided terminations.

The implementation of the FACE Act turned all of these actions into federal crimes, allowing the Department of Justice to charge individuals who damaged clinics, intimidated doctors, patients and staff, or otherwise physically obstructed those attempting to access or offer reproductive health care. But the FACE Act is only as strong as the administration that controls the DOJ, and its willingness to take action. While the Clinton DOJ filed FACE Act charges in four cases, the Republican administration of George W. Bush filed none. Democratic President Barack Obama's DOJ, under Attorney General Eric Holder, filed another seven cases during their eight years in office.[18]

In the first two years of the Trump administration, there were signs that FACE Act enforcement would lag despite an uptick in clinic protests and threats, with charges filed only when they cannot be avoided. Take the case against extreme anti-abortion activist Rusty Thomas, the head of Operation Save America (OSA), and several colleagues, for example. In 2017, OSA arranged an old-fashioned sit-in blockade at EMW Women's Surgical Center in Louisville, Kentucky, the only remaining clinic in the state. The group sat in front of the clinic's front entrance so patients could not enter, refusing to move from their location until police physically removed them. Ten members of the group were later charged with violating the FACE Act.[19] The OSA "rescue" was a blatant attempt to test the new administration's willingness to prosecute anti-abortion activists who were ready to put their religious commitment to ending abortion to the test. The answer—that the DOJ would in fact uphold federal law when pressed—initially looked like a positive response for abortion access supporters. However, the subsequent case of the "Red Rose Rescue" makes the DOJ commitment to upholding and enforcing the FACE Act much less assured.

The "Red Rose Rescues" are spearheaded by Monica Migliorino Miller, a 1980s-era rescuer who used to obtain fetal remains from the dumpsters of abortion clinics in Chicago, creating one of the largest catalogs of post-abortion photographs, which are used as "victim images" by the anti-abortion movement. Unlike the original rescues, where the goal was to stop patients from entering clinics by blocking entrances with their bodies, Red Rose Rescues involve people who go into clinic lobbies, waiting rooms and other areas, where they attempt to pass out red roses with information about crisis pregnancy centers or other avenues for assistance while trying to convince patients not to abort. As with traditional rescues, the Red Rose Rescuers refuse to leave the building under their own efforts, instead going limp once officers arrive on scene, forcing the police to drag their bodies away.[20]

As of March 2019, there had been nearly a dozen Red Rose Rescue attempts in New Mexico, Virginia, Michigan, New Jersey and Maryland, with most of the rescues focused on two Washington DC-area clinics. While there have been multiple arrests and fines—usually for charges like "defiant trespass"—there has yet to be a single FACE Act charge against the group, despite the fact that their specific goal for entering the clinics is to stop people from obtaining abortions.

•

It's now clear that constitutionally protected civil rights and the right to free speech, and the uninhibited religious practice of the religious right, are coming to a head, and that the friction between the two will only grow as social conservatives remain in control of the executive branch. Luckily, there is still the federal courts to stop this power play and ensure that the rights of both parties remain balanced.

Of course, that was before the Trump administration destroyed the judiciary, too.

15

HOW THE RIGHT WON
THE JUDICIARY

AND PREPPED THE PERFECT ABORTION BILL

The sudden death of Justice Antonin Scalia in February 2016 was a turning point for the United States Supreme Court, the significance of which this country is only starting to realize. Prior to Scalia's death, the nine-member Court was more-or-less an evenly divided body, with four reliable liberal votes, four reliable conservative votes, and Justice Anthony Kennedy occupying the role of the coveted "swing vote." With Scalia's death, for the first time in decades, liberals had the chance to shift the balance of power on the Court with a third appointment for President Barack Obama.

Republicans had been able to secure a political advantage during the Obama administration by stymying as many of the president's judicial nominees as possible, and they were not about to let him appoint Scalia's replacement without a fight. On March 16, 2016, Obama nominated DC Circuit Court of Appeals Judge Merrick Garland to replace Scalia. A centrist and well-known figure in legal circles, Garland was viewed as the kind of nominee Republicans couldn't say no to. Except that is exactly what they did. Almost immediately after Garland's nomination was announced, citing an election that was still more than eight months away, Republican Senate Majority Leader Mitch McConnell refused to grant Garland a hearing. McConnell declared that the seat should belong to the next president instead, and that the American public should be allowed to choose which party would fill it. It was a dangerous gambit, but one that paid off for the Republicans.

Grassroots efforts to encourage social conservatives to go to the polls in November 2016 primarily revolved around the idea of keeping Democratic nominee Hillary Clinton from filling the empty Supreme Court seat. According to the *Washington Post's* Philip Bump, an analysis of exit polling data showed that for about 25 percent of Republican voters in 2016, the Supreme Court vacancy was a significant factor in their eventual choice for president, far more than it was for Democratic voters. "Did it make the difference? Trump won thanks to 78,000 voters in three states: Pennsylvania, Wisconsin and Michigan. It is, as we've noted before, a narrow enough margin that a *lot* of things could have made the difference," Bump surmised in June 2018. "But let's answer the question. If the constant emphasis on Supreme Court nominees spurred 78,000 of the 14 million people who cast votes in those states did so to hold a majority on the court, it made the difference. There were about 6.6 million votes cast for Trump in those three states. National exit polls suggest that 1.7 million of them thought that the court was the most important reason to cast that vote."[1]

The Republican voters got exactly what they asked for. Less than two weeks after President Donald Trump was sworn into office, he announced the appointment of Tenth Circuit Court of Appeals Judge Neil Gorsuch to fill the seat left vacant by Republicans' refusal to confirm Garland. Trump chose Gorsuch from a shortlist of potential Supreme Court nominees developed in part by Leonard Leo, the executive vice president of the

Federalist Society, a far-right conservative legal group dedicated to "constitutional originalism" in interpreting laws, and driven to packing the federal judiciary with like-minded judges.

As a nominee, Gorsuch was everything social conservatives could have wanted. He was a graduate of Harvard, Columbia and Oxford, and a former Supreme Court law clerk for then Justice Anthony Kennedy as well as Justice Bryon White. Gorsuch had spent time in the George W. Bush Justice Department before Bush nominated him to the Colorado-based Tenth Circuit. It was while on the Tenth Circuit that Gorsuch joined his colleagues to rule that businesses could bring challenges to the birth control benefit in the Affordable Care Act under the Religious Freedom Restoration Act (RFRA), a federal statute designed to protect religious liberty rights from government overreach. That ruling eventually was appealed and became the 2014 Supreme Court case *Burwell v. Hobby Lobby*, in which the Court ruled 5 to 4 that a "closely held" private corporation was not required to adhere to the Affordable Care Act's requirement for mandatory birth control coverage in their insurance plans because doing so would violate the RFRA.[2]

Gorsuch's could not have been more of a contrast to Garland. Where the Obama selection was a centrist who historically would have been confirmed with wide bi-partisan margins, President Donald Trump's pick was a slap in the face to any attempt at bipartisanship. The left responded as best they could despite lacking the votes to stop Gorsuch's nomination. It took until early April of 2017 for Gorsuch to be confirmed, as Democrats availed themselves of every rule and procedure to slow the confirmation process. McConnell responded by changing the rules. Gorsuch was confirmed 54 to 45, giving him the lowest threshold of support for any successful Supreme Court nominee since Republican President George H. W. Bush appointed Justice Clarence Thomas.

It wasn't a designation he would hold for long, though.

On June 27, 2018, Supreme Court swing vote Anthony Kennedy announced his retirement, providing President Trump with a second seat to fill on the bench, one that would change the make-up of the Court. Replacing the rock-ribbed conservative Judge Scalia with another far-right justice like Gorsuch merely kept the previous Court leanings intact, but adding a second nominee as conservative as Gorsuch or more so to replace Kennedy would move the Court further to the right than it had been since the 1930s.[3]

On July 9, 2018 Trump nominated DC Circuit Court of Appeals Judge Brett Kavanaugh to the now-vacant Kennedy seat and Democrats—knowing that not just abortion rights but marriage equality, voting rights, the separation of church and state, the death penalty and countless other civil rights that Americans have embraced or fought to gain over the last half century were at immediate risk—sprang into action to try and block his nomination.

Kavanaugh, a former clerk for Kennedy, was a well-known Republican operative from the 1990s, when he worked on the special counsel investigation team lead by Kenneth Starr that resulted in the impeachment of Democratic President Bill Clinton. If there was any question that Kavanaugh would be exactly the kind of abortion opponent the anti-abortion movement wanted on the bench, one only had to look at his actions in the case of "Jane Doe," the undocumented minor who sought a termination while in federal custody after crossing the border.

Kavanaugh was one of the two judges on the original three-person panel who denied Doe the right to terminate her pregnancy, even though she had received the needed judicial bypass and had funding to pay for the procedure. When the full DC Circuit reviewed the case and granted Doe the right to leave federal custody to obtain the abortion,

Kavanaugh was one of the judges who dissented, claiming that because Doe wasn't a citizen, and hadn't "properly" entered the United States, she did not have the same right to an abortion afforded to citizens by the US Constitution—and especially not an "abortion on demand," as he put it. It was a statement that his colleague, Judge Patricia Millett, found especially repugnant:

> Abortion on demand? Hardly. Here is what this case holds: a pregnant minor who (i) has an unquestioned constitutional right to choose a pre-viability abortion, and (ii) has satisfied every requirement of state law to obtain an abortion, need not wait additional weeks just because she—in the government's inimitably ironic phrasing—"refuses to leave" its custody, Appellants' Opp'n to Reh'g Pet. 11. That sure does not sound like "on demand" to me. Unless Judge Kavanaugh's dissenting opinion means the demands of the Constitution and Texas law. With that I would agree.[4]

Although Kavanaugh was nominated on July 9, it took nearly three months before he would be sworn in as the next Supreme Court Justice. Confirmation should have been a smooth process since Republicans held a two-vote majority in the Senate, and the death of the filibuster meant that a unified GOP could easily put him in the seat. Instead, his confirmation was marred by repeated credible allegations of sexual misconduct, first by high school acquaintance Christine Blasey Ford, then by a former Yale classmate, Deborah Ramirez. As sexual assault survivors organized at the Capitol to demand a fuller investigation into the allegations, Arizona Republican Senator Jeff Flake, who served on the Judiciary Committee, requested an FBI investigation into the accusations.

However, the investigation remained limited in scope and was given a one-week deadline, with Kavanaugh's nomination continuing forward even as it happened.

Seven days later, the FBI concluded its investigation with a report that was kept private and never released to the public but which, according to the GOP, exonerated Kavanagh. His confirmation was advanced the following day, with a 51 to 49 vote in his favor, and the day after that he was officially confirmed 50 to 48 on a near party-line vote. West Virginia Senator Joe Manchin was the only Democrat to vote to confirm, and Senator Lisa Murkowski of Alaska the only Republican to oppose him (although Murkowski didn't vote on the final confirmation in order to allow a fellow Republican colleague to skip the final vote and attend a wedding instead).[5] Kavanaugh had officially won confirmation—and with the narrowest majority ever for a sitting Supreme Court justice to date.

That bruising battle may have only delayed the inevitable: as long as Republicans had a majority in the Senate, keeping Kavanaugh off the bench was always going to be a near impossibility. What it did do, however, was expose exactly how partisan the newest Supreme Court justice really was. At the height of the confirmation controversy, just when it was unclear exactly how many accounts of sexual misconduct might be pending, Kavanaugh lashed out in his own defense, arguing that not only were all of the allegations false, but that they were obviously a coordinated hit on his professional character orchestrated by the political left. "This whole two-week effort has been a calculated and orchestrated political hit, fueled with apparent pent-up anger about President Trump and the 2016 election, fear that has been unfairly stoked about my judicial record, revenge on behalf of the Clintons and millions of dollars in money from outside left-wing opposition groups," he boldly declared in his sworn testimony, which included the rather ominous warning that "what goes around comes around."[6]

•

If Kavanaugh has a desire to settle scores with the left now that he is ensconced in a lifetime appointment to the highest court in the nation, the time is rapidly approaching. As of April 2019, there were at least twenty cases regarding abortion rights in the legal pipeline, working their way to the Supreme Court for review—and any one of them could provide the opening for a new conservative court majority to overturn *Roe v. Wade* once and for all.

Many of the nearly two dozen cases developed out of the basic set of model bills and restrictions set out in the previous chapters of this book, such as mandatory waiting periods and mandatory ultrasounds, or the exponentially growing body of "heartbeat" abortion bans. Others regard clinic licensing or doctor's privileges that should have been settled under *Whole Woman's Health v. Hellerstedt*, yet are getting a second chance now that the Supreme Court has a more conservative tilt. Another pending case pending involves an Indiana law that makes it a crime to terminate a pregnancy due to the gender, race or potential disability of the embryo or fetus. And one case from Mississippi is a straight no-frills total abortion ban at fifteen weeks—more than a month prior to any possibility of fetal viability.

Yet while all of these cases were possibilities for the ultra-right Roberts court to pick and choose from, there was a new restriction making its way to the front of the line: *Whole Woman's Health, Planned Parenthood Center for Choice, Planned Parenthood of Greater Texas v. Ken Paxton*, a case involving the attempt to ban Dilation and Evacuation (D&E) abortions, based on a model bill that ironically enough had been crafted for Justice Anthony Kennedy.

•

It was just a week before the anniversary of *Roe v. Wade* in 2015 when National Right to Life issued a press release announcing a first of its kind abortion restriction that would be introduced in the state of Kansas. Calling it "a move that will transform the landscape of abortion policy," National Right to Life Director of State Legislation Mary Spaulding Balch effusively praised the "Unborn Child Protection From Dismemberment Act," a new procedural ban that would essentially eliminate the safest, easiest way to perform almost all abortions after the first trimester. Spaulding Balch compared the procedure to the already illegal intact dilation and extraction that had formed the basis of the so-called "partial birth abortion" ban that was challenged in *Gonzales v. Cahart*. She noted repeatedly that Justice Anthony Kennedy had denigrated the process in which a fetus was removed from the uterus, claiming it was "laden with the power to devalue life." According to Spaulding Balch, if Kennedy believed that about an intact D&E, surely he would feel the same about the traditional dilation and evacuation, even if it was done far earlier in a pregnancy, when the fetus was far less mature.[7]

A D&E abortion is commonly used as the primary means of ending a pregnancy after the first trimester. Before about fifteen weeks, abortion can be more easily done using a vacuum aspirator because the embryo or fetus is still small enough that the cannula that is inserted is able to remove it by using pressure, without any other intervention necessary. But once the second trimester begins, the fetus's bones have begun to calcify and are more solid, making it impossible to remove it in one effort. Instead, medical tools like forceps are necessary to remove it in smaller parts, and a curettage and vacuum aspiration is employed at the end to ensure all tissue, placenta and other uterine contents are gone. Otherwise, the pregnant patient would need to be fully dilated and have labor induced in order to terminate. A D&E takes approximately thirty minutes, requires much less dilation, and is a quick and safe medical procedure that can be done in a clinic. An induced labor, on the other hand, can take hours or days, would likely need to be done in a hospital, and can bring greater medical risks to the patient.

But describing a D&E in full detail, like all medical procedures, can be extremely gruesome. And that's exactly what abortion opponents were hoping for when they introduced this specific restriction. The bill banned "knowingly dismembering a living unborn child and extracting such unborn child one piece at a time from the uterus through the use of clamps, grasping forceps, tongs, scissors or similar instruments that, through the convergence of two rigid levers, slice, crush or grasp a portion of the unborn child's body in order to cut or rip it off."[8]

Expert witness, and former abortion provider Dr. Anthony Levatino, explained step by step how a D&E would be performed on a twenty-one week gestation fetus, adding his own political commentary. "Many times a little face will come out and stare back at you. Congratulations! You have just successfully performed a second trimester Suction D&E abortion. You just affirmed her right to choose. If you refuse to believe that this procedure inflicts severe pain on that unborn child, please think again," he told the Kansas Senate Health and Human Services Committee in 2015.[9]

As the ban was debated in the Kansas State Legislature, it became clear that abortion opponents were eager to condemn all abortion— not just D&Es—as emphatically as possible. Leading the charge was Republican State Representative Dick Jones, who managed to work nearly every anti-abortion talking point into his testimony in a house committee hearing. Calling the procedure a "rotten egg" and "a really filthy practice," Jones also suggested tongue in cheek that mothers also be allowed to slaughter their children after birth, then added that abortion was a "holocaust against fetuses." Not content to leave his diatribe in the committee chambers, Jones also informed a reporter that if abortion remained legal, "[W]e're then saying that it's all right to kill quadriplegics because they're a burden on society."[10]

Other than Jones's enthusiastic display of public support, the rest of the bill's progress went mostly unnoticed. The D&E ban rapidly moved through the statehouse and was signed into law on April 7, 2015 by Republican Governor Sam Brownback. Brownback was so overjoyed by this first in the nation restriction that he set out on a state tour to ceremoniously sign the bill over and over again—at a Catholic church "education building" in Lenexa, Kansas, and then at Catholic high schools in the cities of Pittsburg, Hays and Wichita.[11]

In the end, it didn't matter how many times Brownback signed the bill, as the law never actually went into effect in Kansas. In June, a Shawnee County judge blocked the bill before its July implementation, and in December 2015, the Kansas Court of Appeals met to decide whether the preliminary injunction should be extended. On January 22, 2016, the forty-sixth anniversary of *Roe v. Wade*, the judges reached a split decision, which let the lower court's injunction stand, but left the question of whether the state constitution itself suggests there is a right to an abortion unanswered.

By that point, several other states had introduced their own D&E bans, and, like Kansas, had found little success in the courts. As of April 2019, D&E bans have been blocked in Kansas, Oklahoma, Arkansas, Alabama, Ohio, Kentucky, Louisiana and Texas, and have only been enacted in West Virginia and Mississippi, where no one has yet to challenge them in court.[12] Indiana and North Dakota have also passed bans, which also haven't yet been challenged.

Despite the legal failures of D&E bans, it is still likely that one will land before the Supreme Court. Alabama asked the Court to intervene in the fight over its D&E ban, waiting months for the Court to decide whether or not to take action. US District Judge Lee Yeakel ruled Texas's D&E ban unconstitutional in November 2017; the state chose to appeal the decision, sending the case up to the Fifth Circuit, the same circuit which claimed that closing most of the abortion clinics in Texas didn't create an undue burden on the right to terminate a pregnancy, which forced the Supreme Court to step in and reverse that decision in *Whole Woman's Health v. Hellerstedt*.

If any circuit would be eager to reverse a lower court ruling in favor of the right to an abortion, it would be the Fifth. But to date it has not ruled, holding out until the outcome of a different case, *June Medical Services v. Gee,* is resolved. That case is a challenge to a series of Louisiana TRAP laws identical to the ones struck down as unconstitutional in *Hellerstedt,* which could wind up before the Court during the 2019–2020 term. A reversal by the Fifth Circuit would not only allow the Texas ban to take effect, but would also likely force the Supreme Court to step in and resolve the conflict between the Fifth Circuit and the Alabama ban. And abortion opponents are enthusiastically pushing for that to happen sooner rather than later. In February of 2019, twenty-one states' Attorneys General signed an amicus brief urging the Supreme Court to take up Alabama's appeal of their D&E ban injunction, saying they need clarity on states' ability to ban an abortion procedure if there are "safe" alternatives that doctors can use instead:

> The likelihood that such a procedure compromises public respect for life, not to mention the ethics of the medical profession, is unquestionably serious," they write. "Many States would prefer to prohibit the procedure altogether. But in light of applicable precedent, Alabama has instead sought simply to moderate

the dismemberment procedure by requiring that abortion providers use available methods to kill fetuses before dismembering them.[13]

Despite the brief, the Supreme Court announced on June 28, 2019 that it would not take up Alabama's case at this time, leaving the law blocked, at least for now.

Supporters of D&E abortion bans argue that states have the right to restrict procedures that "threaten to erode respect for life," playing for an audience that they originally assumed would be made up of their favorite swing vote, Justice Anthony Kennedy. Now that they have a much more conservative bench to work with, anti-abortion activists could easily switch tactics and put their efforts into convincing the Supreme Court to take up something far more restrictive—like a six-week "heartbeat" ban—instead.

At the same time, congressional lawmakers are hard at work laying the foundation for a proposed federal D&E abortion ban that could eventually make its way to the Supreme Court. Introduced by Republican Senators Mike Rounds of South Dakota and James Lankford of Oklahoma, the "Dismemberment Abortion Ban Act of 2019" will likely never receive the sixty votes it needs to pass the Senate, nor would it get enough support in the House even if it did. What the bill will do, however, is allow Republican Senators to create a congressional record filled with hyperbolic descriptions of limbs torn and skulls being crushed that can be pulled from amicus filings should the Supreme Court finally take up the Alabama appeal.

A D&E ban is in many ways the right's most effective tool for bringing about the end of *Roe v. Wade* because it follows the familiar playbook from *Gonzales* of manipulating discomfort around medical procedures into political opposition against abortion rights. Despite the efforts of abortion foes to block access, close clinics, demonize providers, shame patients who have undergone the procedure and sympathetically humanize embryos, Americans nevertheless remain stubbornly in favor of *Roe v. Wade*, with over 70 percent of respondents as recently as September 2018 saying they wanted the ruling to remain in effect.[14] Abortion opponents simply do not have the public support when it comes to making the procedure illegal, and the only way they can move the needle in their favor is to convince the American public that abortion is grotesque, barbaric, and medically unnecessary. If they can successfully personify the fetus while making the person carrying it an inconsequential afterthought, they may be able to drum up enough political cover to finally ban the procedure completely—even if it is only in a dozen or so states to start. A D&E ban is the perfect vehicle for this quest, as it is in many ways the courtroom version of the graphic fetal imagery being paraded outside abortion clinics across the nation. As anti-abortion activists often say, it's not enough to just make abortion illegal, you have to make it unthinkable as well.

16

WHERE IT ALL ENDS

COMING FULL CIRCLE ON TWENTY-WEEK BANS

If the beginning of the end of *Roe v. Wade* can be traced back to Nebraska and the "Pain-Capable Unborn Child Protection Act" in 2010, it is only fitting that almost ten years later, the Supreme Court may finally be poised to finish the work the Cornhusker State started by taking up another previability abortion ban, this time one billed as a twenty- week "fetal pain" abortion ban.

The spring of 2019 saw an onslaught of extreme previability abortion bans that ranged from eight weeks after the last menstrual period (Missouri—passed) to the moment of fertilization (Alabama—passed), as well as new punishments like life in prison for abortion providers (Alabama—passed), proposed jail time for those who helped a person leave one state to obtain legal abortion care in another (Georgia—passed), even the death penalty for a pregnant person who terminates a pregnancy (Texas—failed). These bills rightfully grabbed the media spotlight, drawing almost universal criticism. But none will ever be enforced, at least not until *Roe* is actually overturned. Meanwhile, the low-key, incremental, no frills ban on abortion at twenty weeks post fertilization continues to plod along under the radar, looking less and less threatening every day. Which is exactly the point of the legislation.

It's that very act of goalpost shifting from the right that could allow Senate Bill 160—the "Pain-Capable Unborn Child Protection Act"—to sail right through Congress without much fuss or fanfare. After all, the difference in twenty-two weeks last menstrual period and the very lowest end of the cusp of viability is little more than a week's difference at most. Does blocking this sort of ban really even matter?

Of course, the answer is yes. Located within the legislation is the anti-abortion movement's end game. First, it lists varying embryonic and fetal development points, and claims that at those points, a fetus or embryo can "feel" pain. The development points range from eight weeks to twenty weeks, with the clear intention of driving the standard for judging these kinds of restrictions away from viability and toward an ever-diminishing gestational point. The idea is to get the Supreme Court to finally move away from viability as a bright line constitutional test. Should the Court take the bait, what started as a twenty-week fetal pain ban will soon become an eight-week ban, and so on and so on as states press to ban abortion far earlier than ever before, upending the trimester framework of *Roe* and the undue burden standard of *Casey* entirely.

How early can this go? The answer is in the federal bill. "After 8 weeks fertilization, the unborn child responds to touch," claims S 160, introduced on January 16, 2019 by South Carolina Republican Senator Lindsey Graham.[1] And if ten weeks after last menstrual period wasn't early enough, anti-abortion policy organization the Charlotte Lozier Institute (an arm of the Susan B. Anthony List) offers research claiming that the "[t]he basic anatomical organization of the human nervous system is established by 6 weeks. The earliest neurons in the cortical brain (the part responsible for thinking, memory, and other higher functions) are established starting at 6 weeks," suggesting that even earlier thresholds for banning abortion that have been rejected by the federal courts as outliers from very conservative states could be on the way back, mainstreamed by Republicans in Congress.[2]

But first, a federal bill needs to make it to the Supreme Court, and on this point abortion opponents are making progress. On April 9, 2019, Senator Graham chaired the Senate hearing for S 160. It was the first major movement on a twenty-week ban at the federal level since Republican women killed the bill in 2015 because it didn't have a well-defined rape exception. Graham didn't let the opportunity go to waste, jumping right in with scientifically suspect claims about fetal pain, saying that "[i]f medical science tells us the baby is well developed at five months, can feel pain . . . then we should have restrictions on abortion. You can only imagine the pain that comes from dismemberment."[3]

Medical science says no such thing, of course. The American College of Obstetricians and Gynecologists (ACOG) states definitively that a fetus is incapable of feeling pain prior to the third trimester. The only ones disputing this fact are the doctors at AAPLOG—the American Academy of Pro-Life Obstetricians and Gynecologists, a 4000-member offshoot of ACOG that is strictly anti-abortion (ACOG boasts an overall membership of about 58,000).[4]

But because only a single medical representative was present on the five-person panel testifying on SB 160, it was AAPLOG's message—and not the one backed by the overwhelming majority of the scientific population—that was advanced in the hearing. "There are small human beings in the womb who are being pulled apart in pieces, or having their skin burned off, or partially delivered through their mothers' vagina and having their brains pierced and sucked out through a suction catheter," testified Donna

Harrison, the executive director of AAPLOG in support of Graham's bill. "The 'Pain-Capable Unborn Child Protection Act' will protect unborn children in the United States from being killed in brutal ways."

Harrison may have been called as a witness in support of the Pain-Capable Unborn Child Protection Act, but it was clear that like the bill itself, the goal of her testimony was to advocate for even more extreme abortion restrictions. Harrison testified that most later gestation abortions are done by either D&E, "partial birth abortion" (Intact D&E) or "saline abortions," despite the fact that intact D&E has already been banned federally since 2007, and saline abortions almost completely disappeared two decades ago once safer, more efficient means of terminating a pregnancy were discovered. Yet Harrison included both of these now historic techniques to reiterate her original argument—that D&E is a "barbaric" procedure that dehumanizes and causes "pain" to a developing fetus.

For the final two minutes of her testimony, Harrison simply recited the same detailed verbal depiction of a D&E abortion that her colleague, Dr. Anthony Levantino, provides when he testifies for legislatures. "If veterinarians ripped apart living dogs and cats to kill them in the same way that living human children are ripped apart in the D&E procedure, the outcry would be deafening," she concluded.[5]

Much like the "Abortion Dismemberment Ban Act of 2019"—the federal D&E ban proposed by Senators Mike Rounds and James Lankford—S 160 uses graphic words and imagery to try and sway public opinion on abortion while also advancing restrictions that can be pushed toward a favorable Supreme Court. It isn't a coincidence that the greatest success the anti-abortion movement has had at the federal level has been with procedural bans, both from a legal and public relations standpoint. And now, if all goes according to the right's plan, the ruling in *Carhart v.*

Gonzales that first opened the door to previability procedure bans won't just provide the language for how to testify in support of restrictions in the most graphic way possible—it will have also given anti-abortion activists the building blocks to reduce, and eventually close entirely, the gestational window for terminating a pregnancy.

Can a twenty-week ban pass on a federal level? It certainly seems like a long shot, as it would require an anti-abortion majority in the House, at least sixty senators who oppose abortion, and a Republican in the White House. As of this moment only one of these criteria have been met, and getting them all in line at the same time may (thankfully) be utterly impossible for the right.

But after nearly a decade where we have seen approximately 400 pieces of individual state based abortion restrictions which have grown even more extreme since the election of President Donald Trump and the seating of two new conservative justices, a federal twenty-week ban may no longer be as far-fetched as it once was. How long will it be before a handful of Democrats decide to use their votes on this bill or a later version as a bargaining chip for securing social security for another decade, or to win someone over to the New Green Deal, for example? After all, abortion became a negotiating point in the battle to pass the Affordable Care Act during the Obama administration. Can we truly expect our supposed allies in congress to stand strong and protect abortion if its tacked onto funding for schools or a Medicaid expansion? Or what if voting for it could prevent a government shutdown? Any of these scenarios could come to play within the next few years, and then we really will see the end of *Roe v. Wade*. And then, after nearly fifty years, the right finally will have won the abortion battle.

NOTES

1: WHERE IT ALL STARTED

1. Interview with Sen. Danielle Conrad, May 20, 2012.

2. Lena H. Sun, "Neb. doctor who performs abortions in Md. Talks about security concerns, future of clinic," *Washington Post*, July 21, 2011, http://www.washingtonpost. com/national/health-science/neb-doctor-who-performs-abortions-in-md-talks-about-security-concerns-future-of-clinic/2011/07/21/gIQAaJMSXI_story.html.

3. Susan J. Lee, JD; Henry J. Peter Ralston, MD; Eleanor A. Drey, MD, EdM; John Colin Partridge, MD, MPH; Mark A. Rosen, MD, "Fetal Pain: A Systematic Multidisciplinary Review of the Evidence," *The Journal of the American Medical Association*, August 24, 2005, http://jama.jamanetwork.com/article.aspx?articleid=201429.

4. The Royal College of Obstetricians and Gynaecologists published their own study in June 2010 that confirmed it was "apparent that connections from the periphery to the cortex are not intact before 24 weeks of gestation and, as most neuroscientists believe that the cortex is necessary for pain perception, it can be concluded that the fetus cannot experience pain in any sense prior to this gestation."

5. "Nebraska Breaks New Ground in Abortion Law With Enactment of LB 1103, Pain Capable Unborn Child Protection Act," Nebraska Right to Life Press Release, 10/15/10, http://www.nerighttolife.org/SiteResources/Data/Templates/t4.asp?docid=571&DocName=PRESS%20RELEASES.

6. JoAnne Young, "Nebraska Legislator Speaker Flood one of Time's '40 under 40,'" *Lincoln Star Journal*, October 14, 2010, http://journalstar.com/news/state-and-regional/govt-and-politics/article_413a86b8-d7f0-11df-88c9-001cc4c03286.html.

7. Martha Stoddard, "State Could Reshape Abortion Policy," *Omaha World Herald*, February 21, 2010, http://www.omaha.com/article/20100221/NEWS01/702219879.

8. Stoddard, "State Could Reshape Abortion Policy."

9. Julie Rovner, "Family At Center of South Dakota Abortion Debate" *NPR*, October 27th, 2008, http://www.npr.org/templates/story/story.php?storyId=95960702.

10. Rovner, "Family At Center of South Dakota Abortion Debate."

11. Keller Russell, "Bill to Limit Abortions After 20 Weeks Draws Testimony From Across Country" *10 11 Now TV*, February 26, 2010, http://www.1011now.com/home/headlines/85374732.

12. Julie Burkhart, "What You Can Do About the Nebraska Abortion Ban that Just Passed," *Huffington Post*, April 13, 2010, http://www.huffingtonpost.com/julie-burkhart/what-you-can-do-about-the_b_535662.

13. JoAnne Young, "Bill to Tighten Abortion Restrictions Gains First-Round Approval," *Lincoln Journal Star*, March 30, 2010 http://journalstar.com/news/local/govt-and-politics/bill-to-tighten-abortion-restrictions-gains-first-round-approval/article_f8ed5360-3b99-11df-b9df-001cc4c03286.

14. Robin Marty, "Nebraska's Legislative Agenda: A Study In Contradictions?" *Rewire.News*, April 12, 2010, https://rewire.news/article/2010/04/12/nebraskas-abortion-legislation-endstretch.

15. "Balancing Faith, Family And Practice: Focus on the Family's Conference For Medical Professionals And Spouses—April 10–12, 2008," http://go.family.org/images/medicalConf/mcBrochure.pdf.

16. Nivedita U Jerath, MD, Chandan Reddy, MD, and Jeffrey S Kutcher MD, "Medical Aspects of the Persistent Vegetative State," *New England Journal of Medicine*, May 26, 1994.

17. Steven Ertelt, "Fetal Pain Abortion Law Takes Effect in Nebraska, Could Set National Trend," *Lifenews*, October 15, 2010, http://www.lifenews.com/2010/10/15/state-5554.

18. Pam Belluck, "Complex Science at Issue in Politics of Fetal Pain," *New York Times*, September 16, 2013, https://www.nytimes.com/2013/09/17/health/complex-science-at-issue-in-politics-of-fetal-pain.html?pagewanted=2&_r=1&hp.

19. Robin Marty, "Nebraska Lawmakers, Seeking to Restrict Abortion Care, Ignore Science, Evidence, and Pleas of Parents," *Rewire.News*, April 2, 2010, https://rewire.news/article/2010/04/02/nebraska-legislature-seeks-restrict-abortion-care-based-faulty-science.

20. Marty, "Nebraska Lawmakers."

21. "Iowa Democrat Predicts Ban on Late-Term Abortion Clinic," Associated Press, May 13, 2011 https://journalstar.com/news/state-and-regional/govt-and-politics/iowa-democrat-predicts-ban-on-late-term-abortion-clinic/article_d164b05d-9690-5869-a9c5-e9f4879a9bd9.html.

22. "Supreme Court Won't Hear Arizona's Appeal on Abortion Ban," *New York Times*, Jan 13, 2014

23. Peter Sullivan, "Court Nixes Idaho Abortion Ban," *The Hill*, May 29, 2015 https://thehill.com/policy/healthcare/243446-court-nixes-idahos-20-week-abortion-ban.

24. "GA Supreme Court rejects challenge to 20 week abortion ban," WABE News, June 19, 2017.

2: OHIO

1. Faith2Action, "Nation's Largest Valentine's Day Delivery to Ohio Statehouse, Thousands of Red-Heart Shaped Balloons to Support Heartbeat Bill!" news release, February 14, 2011.

2. Faith2Action, "Nation's Largest Valentine's Day Delivery to Ohio Statehouse."

3. Aaron Marshall, "Conservative Republicans Relish Their New Power in the Ohio House," *Cleveland Plain Dealer*, January 11, 2011, http://www.cleveland.com/open/index.ssf/2011/01/conservative_cavemen_relish_th.html.

4. Interested Party Testimony on Substitute HB 125 James Bopp Jr.* Ohio Senate Health, Human Services, and Aging Committee December 13, 2011, http://www.ohiosenate.gov/senate2012/Assets/Media/Content/9314.pdf.

5. Alex Stuckey, "'Heartbeat Bill' Divides Ohio Anti-Abortion Leaders," *Columbus Dispatch*, September 27, 2011, http://www.dispatch.com/content/stories/local/2011/09/27/heartbeat-bill-divides-ohio-anti-abortion-leaders.html.

6. Julie Carr Smyth, "Abortion Foes Push Vote on Ohio 'Heartbeat Bill,'" Associated Press, March 29, 2011, http://abclocal.go.com/kfsn/story?section=news/state&id=8041312.

7. Pam Belluck, "Health Experts Dismiss Assertions on Rape," *New York Times*, August 20, 2012, http://www.nytimes.com/2012/08/21/us/politics/rape-assertions-are-dismissed-by-health-experts.html.

8. Peter J. Smith, "Unborn Babies to 'Testify' in Hearing on Ohio Heartbeat Bill," *LifesiteNews*, March 1, 2011, http://www.lifesitenews.com/news/unborn-babies-to-testify-in-hearing-on-ohio-heartbeat-bill.

9. Aaron Marshall, "Ultrasound Images of Two Fetuses Shown to Lawmakers During the 'Heartbeat Bill' Hearing," *Cleveland Plain Dealer*, March 2, 2011, http://www.cleveland.com/open/index.ssf/2011/03/ultrasound_images_of_two_fetus.html.

10. William Hershey, "Commentary: GOP Speaker Must Walk a Tightrope on 'Heartbeat' Bill," *Middletown Journal*, May 15, 2011, http://www.springfieldnewssun.com/news/news/state-regional/commentary-gop-speaker-must-walk-a-tightrope-on--1/nMrWr.

11. Janet Porter, "I can see the end of abortion from here," WorldNetDaily, September 12, 2011, http://www.wnd.com/2011/09/344369.

12. Dr. Lisa Perriera, "Doctor to Ohio Senate: I Do Not Want To Tell My Patients I Cannot Help Them," *Rewire.News*, December 12, 2011, https://rewire.news/article/2011/12/14/doctor-to-ohio-senate-i-do-not-want-to-tell-my-patientes-that-i-cannot-help-them.

13. Interview with Dr. Lisa Perriera, July 23, 2012.

14. Interview with Kellie Copeland, June 12, 2012.

15. Ann Sanner, "Ohio Abortions: Leader Suspends Hearings on Ohio 'Heartbeat' Bill," Associated Press, December 14, 2011, http://www.politico.com/news/stories/1211/70448.html.

16. Marc Kovac, "Kids Want Heartbeat Abortion Bill Passed," *Dix Capital Bureau*, January 11, 2012, http://www.the-daily-record.com/local%20news/2012/01/11/kids-want-heartbeat-abortion-bill-passed.

17. Jim Seigel, "Most Senators Return Anti-Abortion Bears," *The Columbus Dispatch*, January 16, 2012, http://www.dispatch.com/content/stories/local/2012/01/15/most-senators-return-anti-abortion-teddy-bears.html.

18. Laura Bassett, "Anti-Abortion Group Sends Children with Teddy Bears to Lobby Lawmakers," *The Huffington Post*, January 12, 2012, http://www.huffingtonpost.com/2012/01/12/ohio-heartbeat-bill-anti-abortion-group-teddy-bears_n_1202580.html.

19. Copeland interview, June 2012.

20. Blade Columbus Bureau, "'Heartbeat Bill' Backers Send Roses to Ohio Lawmakers," *The Toledo Blade*, February 17, 2012 http://www.toledoblade.com/State/2012/02/17/Bill-s-backers-send-roses-to-Statehouse.html.

21. Newsbrief, "Abortion Foes Ready New Ohio Attack," Associated Press, April 17, 2012, http://www.herald-dispatch.com/news/briefs/x1817470275/AP-NewsBreak-Abortion-foes-ready-new-Ohio-attack.

22. "An Open Letter From Ohio Senate President Tom Niehaus," May 2, 2012, http://www.ohiosenate.gov/senate2012/Assets/Media/Content/9313.pdf.

23. Faith2Action, "Janet Porter Responds to Heartbeat Opponents Quoted in Ohio Senate President's Letter," news release, May 3, 2012 http://www.f2a.org/index.php?option=com_content&view=article&id=2579:janet-porter-responds-to-heartbeat-opponents-quoted-in-ohio-senate-presidents-letter&catid=52:life&Itemid=29.

24. Interview with Dr. Lisa Perriera, July 23, 2012.

25. Planned Parenthood Southwest Ohio Region v. DeWine, Decided October 2, 2012. The panel decision was has appealed to the full Sixth Circuit for consideration and reversal, and in December 2012 the full Sixth Circuit refused reconsideration. Thus, the October 2012 decision stands.

26. Ted Hart, "Heartbeat Bill Supporters Changing Tactics," Ohio Votes.com, June 5, 2012, http://www2.ohio-votes.com/news/2012/jun/05/3/heartbeat-bill-supporters-changing-tactics-ar-1061100.

3: THE END OF MEDICATION ABORTION?

1. Judith Davidoff, "Walker's Budget Removes Insurance Requirement to Cover Birth Control" *Capital Times*, March 02, 2011 http://host.madison.com/news/local/govt-and-politics/walker-s-budget-removes-insurance-requirement-to-cover-birth-control/article_a2f024ee-44d3-11e0-8dc8-001cc4c03286.html.

2. Maggie Fox, "Wisconsin Cuts Funds to Planned Parenthood," *National Journal*, June 26th, 2011, http://www.nationaljournal.com/healthcare/wisconsin-cuts-funds-to-planned-parenthood-20110626.

3. Associated Press, "Walker Signs Slew of Controversial Legislation, Including Anti-Abortion and Sex-Ed Bills," *Wisconsin State Journal*, April 7th, 2012, http://host.madison.com/news/local/govt-and-politics/walker-signs-slew-of-controversial-legislation-including-anti-abortion-and/article_94dab5ec-8008-11e1-a873-001a4bcf887a.html.

4. Associated Press, "Walker Signs Slew of Controversial Legislation, Including Anti-Abortion and Sex-Ed Bills".

5. Monica Davey, "Abortion Drugs Given in Iowa via Video Link," *New York Times*, June 8, 2010, http://www.nytimes.com/2010/06/09/health/policy/09video.html.

6. Michel Martin (Host), "Growing Controversy Surrounds 'Telemed' Abortions," NPR, January 24, 2011, http://www.npr.org/2011/01/24/133182875/Growing-Controversy-Surrounds-Telemed-Abortions.

7. Monica Davey, "Abortion Drugs Given in Iowa via Video Link."

8. Steven Ertelt, "House Votes to Defund Planned Parenthood's Telemed Abortions," *Lifenews*, June 6, 2011, http://www.lifenews.com/2011/06/16/house-votes-to-de-fund-planned-parenthoods-telemed-abortions.

9. U.S. Congress, *Telemedicine Safety Act*, H.R. 5731, 112th Congress, 1st. sess. 2011–2012. introduced in House May 10, 2012, http://www.govtrack.us/congress/bills/112/hr5731/text.

10. Interview with Elizabeth Nash, Guttmacher Institute, July 24, 2012.

11. "Abortion Pill—Fact Not Opinion," Wisconsin Right to Life Website, http://www.wrtl.org/webcam/index.aspx (previously WeAreFactNotOpinion, Youtube, October 22, 2011 http://www.youtube.com/watch?v=x542DALvFos&feature=player_embedded.

12. Todd Richmond, "Wisconsin Assembly debate drags on," Associated Press, March 16, 2012 http://minnesota.publicradio.org/display/web/2012/03/16/wisconsin-assembly-debate.

13. 2011 Wisconsin Act 217, SECTION 10. 253.105(3) http://docs.legis.wisconsin.gov/2011/related/acts/217.

14. Planned Parenthood Advocates of Wisconsin, "Statement from Teri Huyck, President and CEO of Planned Parenthood of Wisconsin, April 20th, 2012," news release, April 20, 2012 http://www.ppawi.org/home/news-media/newsroom/press-releases/PR042012.cmsx.

15. Interview with Dr. Fredrik Broekhuizen, July 25, 2012.

16. Robin Marty, "As Wisconsin Suspends Medical Abortions, One Doctor Explains How the Bill Puts Doctors at Risk," *Rewire.News*, April 23, 2012, https://rewire.news/article/2012/04/23/as-wisconsin-suspends-medication-abortions-one-doctor-explains-how-bill-puts-prof.

17. Robin Marty, "Wisconsin Planned Parenthood to Immediately Stop Offering Medical Abortions Due to New, Medically-Unsupported, Regulations," *Rewire.News*, April 20th, 2012, https://rewire.news/article/2012/04/20/wisconsin-planned-parenthood-to-immediately-stop-offering-medication-abortions-du.

18. Steven Ertelt, "Planned Parenthood Stops Selling Abortion Drug in Wisconsin," *LifeNews.com*, April 20th, 2012 http://www.lifenews.com/2012/04/20/planned-parenthood-stops-selling-abortion-drug-in-wisconsin.

19. Pro-Life Wisconsin, "Planned Parenthood of Wisconsin suspends RU-486 abortions," Pro-Life Wisconsin Website, April 23, 2102 http://www.prolifewisconsin.org/MONUPD_files/April2312monupd.html#article2.

20. NARAL Pro-Choice Wisconsin, "Another Wisconsin Health Provider Ceases

Medication Abortion in Face of Vague New Regulations," news release, May 22nd, 2012 http://www.wispolitics.com/1006/052212NARAL.pdf.

21. Robin Marty, "Planned Parenthood of Wisconsin Sues for Legislative Clarity on Act 217, Calls for End to Practicing Medicine By Legislature," *Rewire.News*, December 12, 2012, https://rewire.news/article/2012/12/12/wisconsin-planned-parenthood-suit-legislative-medicine.

22. Robin Marty, "Planned Parenthood of Wisconsin."

23. Planned Parenthood v. Casey at 877.

24. Planned Parenthood v. Casey at 882.

25. 505 U.S. 833, 884 (1992) (plurality opinion).

26. National Abortion Federation "Safety of Abortion," National Federation of Abortion website, accessed November 23, 2012 http://www.prochoice.org/pubs_research/publications/downloads/about_abortion/safety_of_abortion.pdf.

27. Guttmacher Institute, https://www.guttmacher.org/state-policy/explore/medication-abortion.

28. "Iowa Ban on 'Telemedicine Abortion' Struck Down by State Supreme Court," Associated Press, June 19, 2015.

29. Planned Parenthood Iowa, https://www.plannedparenthood.org/health-center/ia.

30. "Telemed Could Help Fill the Gaps in America's Abortion Care," *Wired*, 8/07/18.

31. Planned Parenthood, *Planned Parenthood Releases New Educational Video on Telemed Abortion*, February 6, 2018.

4: IDAHO

1. Associated Press, "Idaho Woman Charged after Fetus Is Found in a box," *Idaho Press Tribune*, June 1, 2011, http://www.idahopress.com/news/state/article_af96d919-7f3f-5969-8c77-bc918b3cc2b5.html.

2. Brittany Borghi, "Police Find Fetus In Box," LocalNews8.com, Jan 11, 2011, http://www.localnews8.com/news/Police-Find-Fetus-In-Box/-/308662/1562276/-/n4rc04z/-/index.html.

3. Kim Murphy, "Idaho woman's abortion case marks key legal challenge," *L.A. Times*, June 16, 2012, http://articles.latimes.com/2012/jun/16/nation/la-na-idaho-abortion-20120617.

4. Journal Staff, "Woman Accused of Aborting Fetus Will Not Face Charges," *Idaho State Journal*, August 24, 2011.

5. Interview with Dr. Richard Hearn, July 27, 2012.

6. 428 U.S. 106 (1976).

7. Ibid, 108.

8. Ibid, 117.

9. Ibid.

10. McCormack appealed the issue of standing to the 9th Circuit Court of Appeals. Oral arguments were heard on July 9, 2012 and a decision on the issue was expected within six months of that argument. In the meantime, Hearn continues to pursue McCormack's claims on her behalf as a third-party to the litigation.

11. National Advocates for Pregnant Women advances this point in their amicus curiae in the 9th Circuit appeal. "When laws did criminalize abortion, the laws targeted

the third parties who performed unlawful abortions, not the pregnant women themselves, because a primary purpose of these laws was to protect such women from third parties providing dangerous abortions". p. 19 See also e.g., People v. Nixon, 42 Mich. App. 332, 201 N.W.2d 635, 639 (1972) ("The obvious purpose [of the abortion statute enacted in 1846] was to protect the pregnant woman. When one remembers that the passing of the statute predated the advent of antiseptic surgery, the Legislature's wisdom in making criminal any invasion of the woman's person, save when necessary to preserve her life, is unchallengeable.").

12. 428 U.S. 52 (1976).

13. "A Teenager Is Protected from a Forced Abortion" Independence Law Center, Indepencelaw.org, http://independencelaw.org/2012/07/a-teenager-is-protected-from-a-forced-abortion.

14. Robin Marty, "Anti-Choice Activists Applaud 14 year Old Giving Birth," *Rewire.News*, July 25, 2011, https://rewire.news/article/2011/07/25/antichoice-activists-applaud-year-giving-birth.

15. "PA Supreme Court Upholds Respect for Parental Consent," Independence Law Center, Independencelaw.org, http://independencelaw.org/2012/02/pa-supreme-court-upholds-respect-for-parental-consent.

16. States have expanded and contracted this idea with spousal consent requirements, but so far those have not passed constitutional muster.

17. Mike Hixenbaugh, "Ohio Abortion Law Would give Fathers a Say State Legislators Propose Change; Opponents Blast Bill as 'Extreme,'" *Record-Courier*, http://www.record-pub.com/news/article/2327981.

18. U.S. Congress, House, *District of Columbia Pain-Capable Unborn Child Protection Act*, HR 3803, 112th Congress, 1st. sess., , introduced in House July 31, 2012.

19. Kim Murphy, "Idaho Woman's Abortion Case Marks Key Legal Challenge," *Los Angeles Times*, June 16, 2012, http://articles.latimes.com/2012/jun/16/nation/la-na-idaho-abortion-20120617.

20. McCormack v. Hiedeman, Nos. 11-36010,11-36015, September 11, 2012.

21. Ibid.

22. Nancy Hass, "The Next *Roe v. Wade*? An Abortion Controversy in Idaho Inflames Debate," *The Daily Beast*, December 12, 2011, http://www.thedailybeast.com/newsweek/2011/12/11/the-next-roe-v-wade-jennie-mccormack-s-abortion-battle.html.

23. "Court to Hear Appeal of Purvi Patel, Convicted of Feticide," NBC News, May 23, 2016, https://www.nbcnews.com/news/asian-america/court-hear-purvi-patel-feticide-neglect-appeal-n578726.

24. "Murder Charges Dropped Against Georgia Woman Jailed for Taking Abortion Pills," *Washington Post*, June 10, 2015, https://www.washingtonpost.com/news/morning-mix/wp/2015/06/10/woman-charged-with-murder-didnt-have-any-money-to-get-an-abortion-the-legal-way-brother-says/?utm_term=.4dfd9b717bc0.

25. "Woman Who Attempted Coat Hanger Abortion Freed After Pleading Guilty," *Time*, January 12, 2017, http://time.com/4632758/woman-coat-hanger-abortion-anna-yocca-released.

5: INDIANA

1. Ed Pilkington, "Indiana prosecuting Chinese woman for suicide attempt that killed her foetus," *The Guardian*, May 30th, 2012, http://www.guardian.co.uk/world/2012/may/30/indiana-prosecuting-chinese-woman-suicide-foetus.

2. "Premature Birth Complications," American Pregnancy Association, http://www.americanpregnancy.org/labornbirth/complicationspremature.htm.

3. Heather MacWilliams, "Police: Baby Dies After Pregnant Mother Ingests Rat Poison," Fox 59, January 4th, 2011, http://www.chicagotribune.com/news/education/wxin-police-baby-dies-after-pregnan-01032011,0,3796473.story.

4. Jon Murray, "Indiana House OKs Feticide Bill 95–0," *Indy Star*, April 6, 2009, http://www.indystar.com/article/20090406/NEWS05/90406046/Indiana-House-OKs-feticide-bill-95-0.

5. "Infant Dies Days After Pregnant Mom Drank Rat Poison," RTV6–ABC, January 3, 2011, http://www.theindychannel.com/news/infant-dies-days-after-pregnant-mom-drank-rat-poison.

6. RTV6–ABC, January 3, 2011.

7. "Attorney Rips Prosecutor in Infant Rat Poison Death," WRTV Indianapolis, March 16, 2011, http://www.theindychannel.com/news/attorney-rips-prosecutor-in-infant-rat-poison-death.

8. "Doctors Want Charges Dropped in Infant Rat Poison Death," RTV6–ABC, April 1, 2011, http://www.theindychannel.com/news/doctors-want-charges-dropped-in-infant-rat-poison-death.

9. Eleanor Bader, "Criminalizing Pregnancy: How Feticide Laws Made Common Ground for Pro- and Anti-Choice Groups," *TruthOut*, June 14, 2012, http://truth-out.org/news/item/9772-criminalizing-pregnancy-how-feticide-laws-made-common-ground-for-pro-and-anti-choice-groups.

10. Soraya Chemaly, "The United States: Where Pregnancy Is Probationary and Your Body Is a Crime Scene," *Rewire.News*, May 16, 2012, https://rewire.news/article/2012/05/16/united-states-where-pregnancy-is-probationary-and-your-body-is-crime-scene.

11. "Pence, a former federal prosecutor, has argued that Curry never should have pursued the case. She said prosecutors have discretion, and can choose not to press charges in any given case, especially one like Shuai's where there are so many controversial issues. Shuai's case is also the first of its kind in Indiana, she said, so there's no clear precedent for charging a mother with murder based on her actions during pregnancy." Carrie Ritchie, "Murder Charge Raises Women's Rights Questions," *The Indianapolis Star*, January 5, 2013, http://www.usatoday.com/story/news/2013/01/05/infants-death-raises-womens-rights-questions/1566070.

12. Attorney Linda Pence, "The Criminalizing of Pregnancy, *State of Indiana v Bei Bei Shuai*," http://www.pencehensel.com/Briefs/The-Criminalization-of-Pregnancy-State-of-Indiana-v-Bei-Bei-Shuai.pdf.

13. Indiana Code 35-42-1-2, http://www.in.gov/legislative/ic/2010/title35/ar42/ch1.html.

14. "'I Never Said I Didn't Want My Baby': Mom Won't Be Prosecuted" *Des Moines*

Register, February 2, 2010, http://www.momlogic.com/2010/02/i_never_said_i_didnt_want_my_b.php.

15. Gibbs v. State of Mississippi Supreme Court Amicus Briefing, May 20, 2010.

16. Interview, Lynn Paltrow, Executive Director, National Advocates for Pregnant Women, August 10, 2012.

17. Ed Pilkington, "Alone in Alabama, Dispatches from an Inmate Jailed for Her Son's Stillbirth," *The Guardian*, October 7, 2015, https://www.theguardian.com/us-news/2015/oct/07/alabama-chemical-endangerment-pregnancy-amanda-kimbrough.

18. "US Health of Pregnant Women Being Jeopardized by Punitive Laws," Amnesty International, May 23, 2017, https://www.amnesty.org/en/latest/news/2017/05/usa-health-of-pregnant-women-being-jeopardized-by-punitive-laws.

19. Carla Zanoni, Shayna Jacobs, and Ben Fractenberg, "Mother of Fetus Found in Alley Charged with Self-Abortion," *DNAinfo*, Dec 1, 2011, http://www.dnainfo.com/new-york/20111201/washington-heights-inwood/mother-of-fetus-found-alley-charged-with-selfabortion.

20. Interview, Pam Merrit, Reproductive Justice activist, July 22, 2012.

21. Matt Adams, "Plea Deal Reached in Bei Bei Shuai Rat Poison Case" *Fox 59*, August 2, 2013, https://fox59.com/2013/08/02/plea-agreement-reached-in-bei-bei-shuai-case.

6: OKLAHOMA

1. Associated Press, "Oklahoma: Abortion Law Overturned," *New York Times*, August 19, 2009, http://www.nytimes.com/2009/08/19/us/19brfs-ABORTIONLAWO_BRF.html?_r=0.

2. Interview, Michelle Mohaved, Attorney for Center for Reproductive Rights, July 22nd, 2012

3. Amie Newman, "New Oklahoma Law Forces Ultrasounds," *Rewire.News*, April 25, 2008, https://rewire.news/article/2008/04/25/new-oklahoma-law-forces-ultrasounds.

4. Alex Spillius, "Oklahoma Forces Women to Have Ultrasound Before Abortion," *The Telegraph*, April 28, 2010, http://www.telegraph.co.uk/news/worldnews/northamerica/usa/7647166/Oklahoma-forces-women-to-have-ultrasound-before-abortion.html.

5. Interview, Dr. Curtis Boyd, July 24th, 2012.

6. Oklahoma HB 2870 , Section 2.c, https://www.sos.ok.gov/documents/legislation/52nd/2010/2R/HB/2780.pdf.

7. Alabama Code § 26-23A-4 (4);(5).

8. "Woman's Right to Know: States that Offer Ultrasound Option," National Right to Life Committee, January 11, 2012, http://www.nrlc.org/WRTK/UltrasoundLaws/StateUltrasoundLaws.pdf.

9. "Option Ultrasound: Revealing Life to Save Life," Focus on the Family: Be A Voice For Life, http://www.heartlink.org/oupdirectors.cfm.

10. Focus on the Family, "Focus on the Family Clarifies Option Ultrasound

Numbers," October 18, 2011, https://www.focusonthefamily.com/about/newsroom/news-releases/20111018-focus-on-the-family-clarifies-option-ultrasound-numbers.

11. "Focus on the Family—Operation Ultrasound Program, https://www.focusonthefamily.com/pro-life/promos/option-ultrasound-program.

12. "Ultrasound Initiative Guidelines," Knights of Columbus, http://www.kofc.org/un/en/prolife/ultrasound/guidelines.html.

13. Scott Noble, "Life care center dedicates new ultrasound," Minnesota Christian Examiner, October, 2011 http://www.minnesota.christianexaminer.com/Articles/Oct11/Art_Oct11_02.html.

14. Jeanne Monahan, "Ultrasound Policy" Family Research Council, http://www.frc.org/onepagers/ultrasound-policy.

15. Kevin Sack, "In Ultrasound, Abortion Fight Has New Front," New York Times, May 27, 2010, http://www.nytimes.com/2010/05/28/health/policy/28ultrasound.html.

16. "Deception at Crisis Pregnancy Centers, the Crisis Project" Youtube video, http://www.youtube.com/watch?feature=player_embedded&v=b3aH8h3PWHc#!.

17. Tracy Weitz, "Oklahoma Gets Top Pro-Life Honors for Abortion Laws: A Look at Ultrasound," Advancing New Standards In Reproductive Health, January 27, 2011, http://blog.ansirh.org/2011/01/oklahoma-abortion-laws-and-ultrasound.

18. Associated Press, "Hearing Set on Oklahoma Law Suit," NewsOK, April 29, 2010, http://newsok.com/hearing-set-in-planned-parenthood-lawsuit-against-oklahoma/article/3730121.

19. Associated Press, "Judge says Oklahoma cannot force abortion patients to view ultrasound," The Guardian, March 28, 2012, http://www.guardian.co.uk/world/2012/mar/29/abortion-oklahoma-ultrasound-fetus-judge.

20. Barbara Hoberock, "State AG Appeals Court's Ruling Tossing Abortion Ultrasound Bill," Tulsa World, June 22, 2012, http://www.tulsaworld.com/news/article.aspx?subjectid=336&articleid=20120622_16_A1_OKLAHO878149.

21. Corrie MacLaggan, "Texas Senate approves pre-abortion ultrasound law," Reuters, February 17, 2011 http://www.reuters.com/article/2011/02/18/us-texas-abortion-idUSTRE71H03G20110218.

22. Jordan Smith, "Sparks Strikes Again in Abortion Case," Austin Chronicle, August 23, 2011, http://www.austinchronicle.com/blogs/news/2011-08-23/sparks-strikes-again-in-abortion-case.

23. Jodi Jacobson, "Texas sonogram law found to violate the first amendment," Rewire. News, August 30, 2011, https://rewire.news/article/2011/08/30/texas-sonogram-found-violate-first-amendment.

24. Katherine Haenschen, "More on the Mandatory Sonogram Law and Chief Judge Edith Jones," Burnt Orange Report, January 11, 2012, http://www.burntorangereport.com/diary/11715/more-on-the-mandatory-sonogram-law-and-chief-judge-edith-jones.

25. Lakey at 14.

26. Interview, Michelle Mohaved, Attorney for Center for Reproductive Rights, July 22nd, 2012.

27. Interview, Dr. Curtis Boyd, July 24th, 2012.

28. Gretchen S. Stuart, M.D., et al., v. C. Loomis, M.D., et al. 1:11-CV-804, 2014, https://

www.aclu.org/sites/default/files/assets/01.17.14_order_granting_partial_summary_judgment.pdf.

29. Bigelow v. Virginia, 421 U.S. 809 (1975).

30. The Eighth Circuit also has addressed the "compelled speech" issue in Planned Parenthood v. Rounds, setting up another potential conflict of circuits that could prompt Supreme Court review; Casey at 882.

31. Carolyn Jones, "'We Have No Choice': One Woman's Ordeal with Texas' New Sonogram Law," *Texas Observer*, March 15, 2012, http://www.texasobserver.org/we-have-no-choice-one-womans-ordeal-with-texas-new-sonogram-law.

32. "Oklahoma's Mandatory Ultrasound Law Is Ruled Unconstitutional," *Huffington Post*, March 28, 2012 https://www.huffingtonpost.com/2012/03/28/oklahoma-mandatory-ultrasound-law-unconstitutional_n_1386372.html.

33. "Federal Appeals Court Upholds Kentucky Ultrasound Rule," *Louisville Courier Journal*, April 4, 2019, https://www.courier-journal.com/story/news/politics/ky-legislature/2019/04/04/federal-appeals-court-upholds-kentucky-ultrasound-abortion-law/3368859002.

34. "Requirements for Ultrasound," Guttmacher Institute, https://www.guttmacher.org/state-policy/explore/requirements-ultrasound.

7: SOUTH DAKOTA

1. Amanda Robb, "Controversial South Dakota 'Crisis Pregnancy Center' Activist Leslee Unruh," *More Magazine*, April 6, 2010, http://www.more.com/news/womens-issues/leslee-unruhs-facts-life.

2. Andy Kospa, "Alpha Center and their $2 million government grant," *Off The Record: On Religion, Politics and Equality*, March 23, 2011, http://akopsa.wordpress.com/2011/03/23/south-dakotas-anti-abortion-law-cpc-djour-alpha-center-and-their-2-million-government-grant.

3. Angela Kennecke, "Pro-choice Groups Fight Abortion Ban Proposal," Keloland Television, March 12, 2008 http://www.keloland.com/newsdetail.cfm/pro-choice-group-fights-abortion-ban-proposal/?id=0,67375.

4. South Dakota HB 1217, http://legis.state.sd.us/sessions/2011/Bill.aspx?File=H-B1217ENR.htm.

5. Nancy Gibbs, "When Is an Abortion Not an Abortion?" *Time*, March 6, 2006, http://www.time.com/time/nation/article/0,8599,1170368,00.html.

6. Gibbs, "When is an abortion not an abortion?"

7. Interview, Alisha Sedor, Executive Director NARAL Pro-Choice South Dakota, July 22, 2012.

8. Interview, Sunny Clifford, Lakota Reproductive Rights Advocate.

9. South Dakota HB 1217, February 12, 2011.

10. South Dakota HB 1217, February 12, 2011.

11. Sofia Resnick, "Taxpayer-Funded Crisis Pregnancy Centers Using Religion to Oppose Abortion," *The American Independent*, April 24th, 2012, http://www.huffingtonpost.com/2012/04/24/abortion-religion-pregnancy-centers_n_1446506.html.

12. Robin Marty, "Will Draconian South Dakota Force Women to Visit Religious

Pregnancy Centers Before Abortions?" Alternet, February 18, 2011, http://www.alternet.org/story/149969/will_draconian_south_dakota_force_women_to_visit_religious_pregnancy_centers_before_abortions?page=0%2C2&paging=off.

13. Rob Boston, "Pregnant Pause: Taxpayer Funding for Abortion 'Counseling' Subsidizes Fundamentalist Religion," Americans United, March 31, 2011, https://www.au.org/blogs/wall-of-separation/pregnant-pause-taxpayer-funding-for-abortion-counseling-subsidizes.

14. Mary Garrigan, "Pregnancy Centers Wait Out Daugaard's Decision," Rapid City Journal, March 17, 2011, https://rapidcityjournal.com/news/pregnancy-centers-wait-out-daugaard-s-decision/article_cab7966e-5032-11e0-a45b-001cc4c002e0.html.

15. Mary Garrigan, "Pregnancy Centers Wait Out Daugaard's Decision."

16. Kristen Gosling, "Governor signs 3-day wait for abortion into law," Associated Press, March 22, 2011, https://siouxcityjournal.com/news/state-and-regional/south-dakota/south-dakota-governor-signs--day-wait-for-abortion-into/article_b69936fe-54a3-11e0-9389-001cc4c03286.html.

17. Kristen Gosling, "Governor signs 3-day wait for abortion into law."

18. Robin Marty, "Just Who Is Paying to Defend Anti-Choice Laws in South Dakota?" Rewire.News, March 27, 2011, https://rewire.news/article/2011/03/27/mysterious-money-south-dakota-abortion-will-cost-state-either.

19. Robin Marty, "Patron of Live Action Films Among Contributors to Defense of South Dakota's Newest Anti-Choice Bill," Rewire.News, March 28th, 2011, https://rewire.news/article/2011/03/28/patron-lila-roses-live-action-films-among-those-paying-defense-south-dakotas-newest-antichoice-bill.

20. Robin Marty, "Patron of Live Action Films Among Contributors to Defense of South Dakota's Newest Anti-Choice Bill."

21. Robin Marty, "Planned Parenthood, ACLU Sue South Dakota Over New Abortion Restrictions," Rewire.News, May 27, 2011, https://rewire.news/article/2011/05/27/planned-parenthood-aclu-sues-south-dakota-over-unconstitutional-abortion-access-laws.

22. John Terbush, "Planned Parenthood Sues South Dakota Over Abortion Law," Talking Points Memo, May 28, 2011, http://tpmmuckraker.talkingpointsmemo.com/2011/05/planned_parenthood_sues_south_dakota_over_restrict.php.

23. Jodi Jacobson, "Court Blocks Anti-Choice Legislation in South Dakota," Rewire.News, June 30, 2011, https://rewire.news/article/2011/06/30/court-blocks-antichoice-legislation-south-dakota-0.

24. Mary Garrigan, "Crisis Pregnancy Centers Enter Suit Over State Anti-Abortion Law," Rapid City Journal, January 17, 2012, http://rapidcityjournal.com/news/crisis-pregnancy-centers-enter-suit-over-state-anti-abortion-law/article_9041b29e-40d7-11e1-8729-0019bb2963f4.html.

25. Casey at 882.

26. Planned Parenthood v. Rounds, 530 F.3rd 724 (8th Cir. 2008).

27. Ibid.

28. Ibid at 26, quoting Gonzales, 550 U.S. at 163.

29. Wheeldon v. Madison, 374 N.W.2d 367, 375 (S.D. 1985).

30. Rounds at 14 citing Brenda Major et al., American Psychological Association, Report of the APA Task Force on Mental Health and Abortion 68 (2008).

31. Planned Parenthood v. Rounds, Nos. 09-3231/3233/3262 (July 24, 2012).

32. Ibid, 14.

33. Jodi Jacobson, "Journal Considering Retraction of Article Used to Support Federal Court Ruling on South Dakota Law," Rewire.News, June 25, 2012, https://rewire.news/article/2012/07/25/researchers-urge-retraction-by-journal-article-used-to-support-federal-court-ruli.

34. Interview, Heather Stringfellow, Vice President of Public Policy at the Planned Parenthood Action Council of Utah, July 24, 2012.

35. "Planned Parenthood: We Continue to Fight for our Patients," Planned Parenthood Minnesota, North Dakota, South Dakota, December 21, 2012, http://www.plannedparenthood.org/about-us/newsroom/local-press-releases/planned-parenthood-we-continue-fight-our-patients-40730.htm.

36. "How long do CPCs Need for Counseling? In South Dakota, a Really Long Time," Rewire.News, February 24, 2013, https://rewire.news/article/2013/02/24/exactly-how-long-do-cpcs-need-for-counseling-in-south-dakota-a-reeaally-long-time.

37. "Missouri Lawmaker Compares Getting Abortion to Buying Carpeting," UPI, April 9, 2014, https://www.upi.com/Top_News/US/2014/04/09/Mo-lawmaker-compares-getting-abortion-to-buying-carpeting/1831397072675.

38. "Missouri Governor Eric Greitens Resigns," The Two-Way, May 29, 2018 https://www.npr.org/sections/thetwo-way/2018/05/29/615295346/missouri-gov-eric-greitens-resigns.

8: WASHINGTON, DC

1. Carolyn Dryer, "Groups Protest Franks Anti-Abortion Bill," Glendale Star, March 15, 2012, http://www.glendalestar.com/news/headlines/article_730c1366-6d48-11e1-894d-0019bb2963f4.html.

2. Laura Bassett, "Trent Franks, Arizona Congressman, Targets D.C. Abortion Rights," Huffington Post, May 16, 2012, http://www.huffingtonpost.com/2012/05/16/trent-franks-dc-abortion-rights_n_1521667.html.

3. Interview, Gloria Feldt, July 25, 2012.

4. "DC Abortion Ban Lifted by House of Representatives: Effort Moves to Senate," Rewire.News, July 17, 2009, https://rewire.news/article/2009/07/16/dc-abortion-ban-lifted-house-representatives-effort-moves-senate.

5. The ban is not automatic but enacting it is usually one of the first things Republicans do when they take over the House, either by introducing it as a standalone bill or tacking it on to some other bill.

6. Congresswoman Eleanor Holmes Norton, "Norton Urges President to Not Allow D.C. to Be Used as Bargaining Chip in CR Negotiations," March 29, 2011, http://www.norton.house.gov/index.php?option=com_content&task=view&id=2056&Itemid=99999999.

7. Sabrina Tavernise, "Abortion Limit Is Renewed, as Is Washington Anger," New York

Times, April 10, 2011, http://www.nytimes.com/2011/04/11/us/politics/11district. html?_r=0.

8. Interview, Val Vilott, executive director, DC Abortion Funds, July 27, 2012.

9. "State Funding of Abortion Under Medicaid," Guttmacher Institute, https://www. guttmacher.org/state-policy/explore/state-funding-abortion-under-medicaid.

10. Robin Marty, "A Minnesota Decision Shows Every Woman Has the Right to Choose," *Rewire.News*, June 7, 2010, https://rewire.news/article/2010/06/07/minnesotans-gomez-shows-every-woman-right-choose.

11. "Are You in the Know? Abortion Costs in the United States," Guttmacher Institute, http://www.guttmacher.org/in-the-know/abortion-costs.html.

12. "Clash Over Abortion Stalls Health Care Bill Again," National Public Radio, March 21, 2018 https://www.npr.org/sections/health-shots/2018/03/21/595191785/clash-over-abortion-hobbles-a-health-bill-again-here-s-how.

13. Elizabeth Aguilera, "Trump's Under the Radar $1 Abortion Bill Idea," *Mercury News*, March 5, 2019 https://www.mercurynews.com/2019/03/04/trumps-under-the-radar-1-abortion-bill-idea.

14. "How Can I Find All of the Money I Need?" National Network of Abortion Funds, http://www.fundabortionnow.org/get-help/financial-counseling.

15. "Restrictions on Medicaid Funding for Abortions: A Literature Review," Guttmacher Institute, 2009, http://www.guttmacher.org/pubs/MedicaidLitReview.pdf.

16. 42 U.S.C. §§ 1396a(a)(13)(B) (1970 ed., Supp. V), 1396d(a)(1)-(5) 91970 ed. and Supp. V).

17. 42 U.S.C. § 1396a(a)(17) (1970 ed., Supp. V).

18. 3 Penn. Bulletin 2207, 2209 (September 29, 1973).

19. Beal, 432 U.S. at 445.

20. Ibid.

21. Ibid. (summarizing plaintiffs' arguments).

22. Beal, 432 U.S. at 445.

23. Ibid.

24. Beal, 432 U.S. at 444.

25. Ibid, 444–45 (emphasis in original).

26. Ibid, 470 (summarizing plaintiffs' argument).

27. Maher, 432 U.S. at 469.

28. Ibid, 469–70.

29. Maher, 432 U.S. at 470–71.

30. Ibid, 471.

31. Maher, 432 U.S., 478 (citation and internal quotation marks omitted).

32. Ibid (quoting *Roe*, 410 U.S. at 162-63); Ibid.(quoting Beal v. Doe, 432 U.S. 438, 446 (1977).

33. Ibid, 478–79.

34. Ibid, 479.

35. Ibid, 483.

36. Zbaraz v. Quern, 469 F.Supp. 1212, 1221 (N.D. Ill. 1979).

37. Williams v. Zbaraz, 448 U.S. at 369.

38. Abortion rates by income, Guttmacher Institute. https://www.guttmacher.org/infographic/2017/abortion-rates-income.

39. Women's Medical Fund, Stories, http://womensmedicalfund.org/index.php/stories.

40. "Emergency Funding Request, Woman with Multiple Cancers Needs Your Help," New York Abortion Access Fund, June 7, 2012, http://www.nyaaf.org/2012/06/emergency-funding-request-woman-with-multiple-cancers-needs-your-help.

41. Associated Press, "Abortion Insurance Bill Dies in Washington Senate," The Columbian, March 2, 2012, http://www.columbian.com/news/2012/mar/02/abortion-insurance-bill-dies-in-wash-senate.

42. "Insurance Plans that Cover Pregnancy Must also Cover Abortion under New Washington Law," Q13 Fox News, March 21, 2018, https://q13fox.com/2018/03/21/insurance-plans-that-cover-pregnancy-must-also-cover-abortions-under-new-washington-law.

43. Congresswoman Eleanor Holmes Norton, "Statement of Congresswoman Eleanor Holmes Norton on H.R. 3, the No Taxpayer Funding for Abortion Act," House Committee on the Judiciary Subcommittee on the Constitution, February 8, 2011, http://www.norton.house.gov/index.php?option=com_content&task=view&id=1994&Itemid=88.

44. Katie Rogers, "Trent Franks, Accused of Offering $5 Million to Aide for Surrogacy, Resigns," New York Times, December 8, 2017, https://www.nytimes.com/2017/12/08/us/politics/trent-franks-sexual-surrogacy-harassment.html.

9: TEXAS

1. Governor Rick Perry, "Prepared Remarks for 'Light of Life Dinner and Gala,'" September 26, 2009, http://governor.state.tx.us/news/speech/13747.

2. Danielle Connolly, "Shelby Commission votes for family-planning contract with Christ Community," The Commercial Appeal, October 11, 2011, http://www.commercialappeal.com/news/2011/oct/17/shelby-county-commission-votes-family-planning-con.

3. Robin Marty, "Planned Parenthood Greater Memphis Region Receives $395,000 Title X Grant to Make Up for Funds Given to Religious Health Group," Rewire.News, July 5, 2012, https://rewire.news/article/2012/07/05/planned-parenthood-greater-memphis-region-receives-395000-title-x-grant-to-make-u.

4. Robin Marty, "Ohio Republicans Attempting to Defund Planned Parenthood, Give Money to Groups that Don't Provide Birth Control," Rewire.News, April 17, 2011, https://rewire.news/article/2012/04/17/ohio-republicans-attempting-to-defund-planned-parenthood.

5. "The Uninsured In Texas, " Texas Medical Association, http://www.texmed.org/Uninsured_in_Texas.

6. "The Uninsured In Texas, " Texas Medical Association, http://www.texmed.org/Uninsured_in_Texas.

7. Interview, Veronica Bayetti Flores, Policy Research Specialist at the National Latina Institute for Reproductive Health, July 27th, 2012.

8. Adam Thomas, "Policy Solutions for Preventing Unplanned Pregnancies,"

Brookings Institute, March 2012 http://www.brookings.edu/research/reports/2012/03/unplanned-pregnancy-thomas.

9. Pam Belluck and Emily Ramshaw, "Texas Women's Clinics Retreat as Finances Are Cut," *New York Times*, March 7, 2012, http://www.nytimes.com/2012/03/08/us/texas-womens-clinics-retreat-as-finances-are-cut.html?pagewanted=all&_r=0.

10. Belluck and Ramshaw, "Texas Women's Clinics."

11. Belluck and Ramshaw, "Texas Women's Clinics."

12. Belluck and Ramshaw, "Texas Women's Clinics."

13. Belluck and Ramshaw, "Texas Women's Clinics."

14. Jordan Smith, "Rick Perry's War on Women," *The Nation*, December 19, 2011, http://www.thenation.com/article/164880/rick-perrys-war-women#.

15. Patrick Brendel, "State Abortion-Alternatives Program Funds Christian Nonprofits in Houston," *Washington Independent*, March 15, 2011 http://americanindependent.com/174776/texas-anti-abortion-programserves-fewer-clients-than-targeted.

16. Editorial, "Rick Perry: Women's Health vs. Abortion Politics," *Abilene Reporter News*, March 12, 2012, http://www.reporternews.com/news/2012/mar/08/rick-perry-womens-health-vs-abortion-politics.

17. "Gov. Perry Pledges State Will Take Care of Texas Women if Obama Administration Ends Women's Health Program Funding, as Threatened," Office of the Governor Rick Perry, March 8, 2012, http://governor.state.tx.us/news/press-release/17020.

18. Texas Catholic Conference, "Texas Bishops Support True, Comprehensive Women's Health Programs http://www.txcatholic.org/the-church-in-texas/134-texas-bishops-support-true-comprehensive-womens-health-program.

19. Interview, Jon O'Brien, President of Catholics for Choice, August 7, 2012.

20. Andrea Grimes, "All Those Alternatives to Planned Parenthood? In Texas, At Least, They Don't Exist," *Rewire.News*, April 5th, 2011, https://rewire.news/article/2011/04/05/where-will-health-care-when-family-planning-funds-thing-past.

21. Planned Parenthood, "Federal Judge in Texas Rules in Favor of Women's Health," April 30, 2012, http://www.plannedparenthood.org/about-us/newsroom/press-releases/federal-judge-texas-rules-favor-womens-health-39241.htm.

22. "Texas' Department of Health and Human Services Letter to Fifth Circuit Court of Appeals," July 10, 2012, http://www.ca5.uscourts.gov/opinions/pub/12/12-50377-CV0.wpd.pdf.

23. Hollie O'Connor, "Medical Groups Oppose Women's Health Program Rule," *The Texas Tribune*, August 6, 2012, http://www.texastribune.org/2012/08/06/tma-rejects-rule-banning-discussion-abortion.

24. "Governor's Letter to HHS Secretary Kathleen Sebelius," July 9, 2012, http://governor.state.tx.us/files/press-office/O-SebeliusKathleen201207090024.pdf.

25. 42 U.S.C. § 300(a).

26. 53 Fed. Reg. 2923-24 (1988).

27. Ibid.

28. Ibid, § 59.8(a)(3).

29. Ibid, § 59.8(b)(5).

30. 42 CFR § 59.10(a).

31. Ibid.

32. 42 CFR § 59.9.

33. Ibid.

34. Rust v. Sullivan, 500 U.S.183 (1991).

35. *Rust*, 500 U.S. at 183-91.

36. *Rust*, 500 U.S. at 192.

37. Ibid, 194.

38. *Rust*, 500 U.S. at 196.

39. Ibid.

40. Ibid.

41. 516 U.S., 476.

42. Carolyn Jones, "One Year Later, Cuts to Women's Health Have Hurt More Than Just Planned Parenthood," *Texas Observer*, August 15, 2012, http://www.texasobserver.org/one-year-later-cuts-to-womens-health-have-hurt-more-than-just-planned-parenthood.

43. Jones, "One Year Later, Cuts to Women's Health Have Hurt More Than Just Planned Parenthood."

44. Brianna Stone, "Anti-abortion group was awarded millions but only helped 5 percent of the 70,000 it vowed to serve," *Dallas Morning News*, September 26, 2018, https://www.dallasnews.com/business/health-care/2018/09/26/anti-abortion-group-awarded-millions-failed-serve-thousands-low-income-women-promised.

45. Jeremy Blackman, "Texas gave anti-abortion group millions for women's health, despite warnings," *Houston Chronicle*, February 25, 2019, https://www.houston-chronicle.com/news/politics/texas/article/Texas-gave-anti-abortion-group-millions-for-13638235.php.

46. Kinsey Hasstedt, "Recent funding restrictions on the U.S. family planning safety net may foreshadow what's to come," *Guttmacher Policy Review*, December 19, 2016, https://www.guttmacher.org/gpr/2016/12/recent-funding-restrictions-us-family-planning-safety-net-may-foreshadow-what-come.

47. Alice Miranda Ollstein, "Appeals court rules Ohio can defund Planned Parenthood," *Politico*, March 12, 2019, https://www.politico.com/story/2019/03/12/defund-planned-parenthood-ohio-lawsuit-1262052.

48. On August 21, 2012, the Fifth Circuit held in Planned Parenthood v. Suehs that the Texas rule defining abortion affiliate to include any clinic tied to Planned Parenthood, regardless if they performed abortions, and cutting off state and federal grant money to those clinics could be implemented.

49. Pam Belluck, "Trump Administration Blocks Funds for Planned Parenthood and Others Over Abortion Referrals," *New York Times*, February 22, 2019, https://www.nytimes.com/2019/02/22/health/trump-defunds-planned-parenthood.html.

10: KANSAS

1. Michael Clancy, "Nun at St. Joseph's Hospital rebuked over abortion to save woman," *Arizona Republic*, May 19, 2010, http://www.azcentral.com/news/articles/2010/05/15/20100515phoenix-catholic-nun-abortion.html.

2. St. Joseph's Hospital and Medical Center, "St. Joseph's Statement Regarding

the Bishop's Announcement," http://www.stjosephs-phx.org/Who_We_Are/Press_Center/211990.

3. Associated Press, "Arizona Hospital Loses Status over Abortion Case," *USA Today*, December 22, 2010, http://usatoday30.usatoday.com/news/religion/2010-12-21-phoenix-catholic-hospital_N.htm.

4. American Civil Liberties Union, "ACLU Asks Government to Ensure That Religiously-Affiliated Hospitals Provide Emergency Reproductive Health Care," July 1, 2010, http://www.aclu.org/reproductive-freedom/aclu-asks-government-ensure-religiously-affiliated-hospitals-provide-emergency.

5. Data from Catholic Healthcare in the United States, https://www.chausa.org/about/about/facts-statistics, and Americans United for the Separation of Church and State, "Religiously Affiliated Hospitals," https://www.au.org/issues/religiously-affiliated-hospitals.

6. This is the paradox created by *Casey*. Since, according to *Casey*, women do not have an absolute right to terminate a pregnancy prior to viability because even then the state retains some interest in promoting potential fetal life, an abortion restriction may be "particularly burdensome" on women by creating an increase in cost and potential delays, and still not create an "undue burden" on that right to terminate a pregnancy.

7. See generally Hobby Lobby Stores v. Sebelius, O'Brien v. HHS, Legatus v. Sebelius, and Autocam Corp. v. Sebelius, all of which are pending in U.S. Courts of Appeals.

8. See generally ACLU, *Conflicts Between Religious Refusals and Women's Health: How the Courts Respond* (2002) for the spectrum of religious refusal lawsuits and constitutional arguments and the shifting legal landscape reflected in opinions such as Shelton v. Univ. of Med & Dentristy, 223 F 3d 220 (3rd Cir 2000) and Valley Hosp. Ass'n Inv. v. Mat-Su Coal. for Choice, 948 P2d 963, 972 (Alaska 1997).

9. On The Issues, "Sam Brownback on Abortion" http://www.ontheissues.org/social/Sam_Brownback_Abortion.htm.

10. On the Issues, "Sam Brownback on Abortion."

11. Interview, Meghan Smith, State Coordinator Catholics for Choice, August 3, 2012.

12. Steven Kreytak, "Bus driver who refused to take woman to Planned Parenthood gets $21K in settlement," *Austin American Statesman*, April 25, 2011, http://www.statesman.com/blogs/content/shared-gen/blogs/austin/courts/entries/2011/04/25/driver_who_refused_to_bring_wo.html.

13. Kathleen Gilbert, "Interview: Bus Driver Fired For Refusing to Drive Woman To Abortion Clinic," *Lifesite*, July 20, 2010, http://www.lifesitenews.com/news/archive//ldn/2010/jul/10072008.

14. Seth Augenstein, "12 Nurses Accuse UMDNJ of Forcing Them to Assist in Abortion Cases Despite Religious and Moral Objections," *New Jersey Star Ledger*, November 14, 2011, http://www.nj.com/news/index.ssf/2011/11/12_nurses_accuse_umdnj_of_forc.html.

15. George Prentiss, "Planned Parenthood: Walgreens Pharmacist Refused to Fill

Prescription," *Boise Weekly*, January 12, 2011, http://www.boiseweekly.com/CityDesk/archives/2011/01/12/planned-parenthood-walgreens-pharmacist-refused-to-fill-presciption.

16. George Prentiss, "No Law Requires a Pharmacist to Fill a Prescription," *Boise Weekly*, January 24, 2011, http://www.boiseweekly.com/CityDesk/archives/2011/01/24/no-law-requires-pharmacist-to-fill-a-prescription.

17. Interview, Jon O'Brien, President, Catholics for Choice, August 3, 2012.

18. Stephen Webster, "Kansas Republicans Look to Profit Off Abortion Taxes," *Raw Story*, March 9, 2012, http://www.rawstory.com/rs/2012/03/09/kansas-republicans-look-to-profit-off-abortion-taxes.

19. Brad Cooper, "Kansas House Advances 'Conscience' Protection for Drugs that Might Cause Abortion," *Kansas City Star*, March 28, 2012, http://www.kansascity.com/2012/03/28/3520963/kansas-house-agrees-to-extends.html.

20. Interview, Holly Weatherford, ACLU Kansas, August 8, 2012.

21. Food And Drug Administration: Ella Labeling Information, http://www.accessdata.fda.gov/drugsatfda_docs/label/2010/022474s000lbl.pdf.

22. Pam Belluck, "Abortion Qualms on Morning-After Pill May Be Unfounded," *New York Times*, June 5, 2012, http://www.nytimes.com/2012/06/06/health/research/morning-after-pills-dont-block-implantation-science-suggests.html?pagewanted=all&_r=0.

23. Interview, Dr. Gabrielle Goodrick, July 29, 2012.

24. Marimer Matos, "Rape Victim Can Sue for Denied Contraception," *Courthouse News*, June 25, 2012, http://www.courthousenews.com/2012/06/25/47785.htm.

25. Michael Winter, "Anti-Abortion Group Obtains Kansas Clinic Records from Trash," *USA Today*, May 4, 2012, http://content.usatoday.com/communities/ondeadline/post/2012/05/anti-abortion-group-obtains-kansas-clinic-records-from-trash/1#.UQOdueim5e4.

26. Donald Bradley and Alan Baverly, "Kansas Investigates Operations Rescues's Child Sexual Abuse Claim Against Abortion Clinic," *Kansas City Star*, May 4, 2012, http://www.mcclatchydc.com/2012/05/04/v-print/147705/kansas-investigates-operation.html.

11: ARIZONA

1. Rachel Gold and Elizabeth Nash, "Another Busy Year: State Legislative Trends on Reproductive Health and Abortion in 2009," *Rewire.News*, January 21, 2010, https://rewire.news/article/2010/01/21/another-busy-year-state-legislative-trends-reproductive-health-and-abortion-2009.

2. Interview, Veronica Bayetti Flores, Policy Research Analyst for the National Latina Institute for Reproductive Health, August 2, 2012.

3. E.J. Montini, "Legislature, Anti-Abortion and Anti-Child," *Arizona Republic*, July 7, 2011, http://www.azcentral.com/arizonarepublic/local/articles/2011/07/07/20110707Montini0707.html.

4. Betsy Russell, "Closing Debate: Winder Compares Abortion to U.S. War Casualties," *Idaho Spokesman*, March 19, 2012, http://www.spokesman.com/blogs/boise/2012/mar/19/closing-debate-winder-compares-abortion-us-war-casualties.

5. Evan Wyloge, "Arizona Bill Would Prevent 'Wrongful Birth' Lawsuits," *AZ Capitol Times*, February 8, 2012, http://azcapitoltimes.com/news/2012/02/08/bill-would-prevent-wrongful-birth-lawsuits.

6. Interview, Dr, Gabrielle Goodrick, July 28, 2012.

7. Jessica Mason Pieklo, "Anti-Choice Medical Malpractice Shields Threaten to Permanently Alter Medical Care for Women," *Rewire.News*, April 5, 2012, https://rewire.news/article/2012/04/05/medical-malpractice-shields-threaten-to-permanently-alter-medical-care-women.

8. To be extra sure that doctors in Arizona understood their directive was to coerce women out of having an abortion, the state passed SB 1365. SB 1365 prohibits the state from denying, revoking, or suspending a professional or occupational license based on any action deriving from a person's religious convictions. It's a broad expansion of the state's conscience clause that already allows pharmacists, doctors, or other health care workers to refuse to perform abortions or to prescribe emergency contraception (though it is contraception, not an abortifacient) based on religious objections. Now, any licensed professional can deny services to anyone by declaring that their "sincerely held" religious belief is in conflict with otherwise prohibited and discriminatory conduct and be insulated from professional repercussions for doing so. That means, for example, that attorneys can now decline to represent health care workers facing complaints related to the delivery of reproductive health care, or they can refuse to represent an individual simply because she happens to be gay. See https://rewire.news/article/2012/05/20/arizona-law-endorses-malpractice-and-discrimination-in-defense-religious-liberty.

9. HB 2036 Women's Health and Safety Act Fact Sheet, Center for Arizona Policy, January, 2012.

10. "Dr. Isaacson Letter to Senate President and House Speaker re H.B. 2036, March 7, 2012.

11. "Center for Reproductive Rights, ACLU Launch New Legal Challenge to Block Arizona's Cruel, Unconstitutional Abortion Ban," Center for Reproductive Rights, July 12, 2012, http://reproductiverights.org/en/press-room/center-for-reproductive-rights-aclu-launch-new-legal-challenge-to-block-arizonas-cruel-un.

12. "Anti-Abortionists on Trial," *New York Times*, July 25, 2012, http://www.nytimes.com/2012/07/26/opinion/anti-abortionists-on-trial.html?_r=2&ref=opinion.

13. Order p. 9 of 15.

14. See Gonzales, 550 U.S. at 157-58 ("the fact that a law which serves a valid purpose, one not designed to strike at the right itself, has the incidental effect of making it more difficult or more expensive to procure an abortion cannot be enough to invalidate it.") (quoting Roe v. Wade, 505 U.S. at 874), 11.

15. Robin Marty and Jessica Mason Pieklo, "Goodbye, Trimesters: How The Arizona Court Ruling May Turn Roe On Its Head," *Rewire.News*, July 31, 2012, https://rewire.news/article/2012/07/31/good-bye-trimesters-how-arizona-court-ruling-will-turn-roe-on-its-head.

16. Ayotte v. Planned Parenthood, 546 U.S. 320 (2006)

17. *Ayotte*, 546 U.S. at 328-29 (citing cases).

18. Parties briefs to the court are due in the fall of 2012 with arguments to be scheduled from there. A ruling in the case would follow several months from there.

19. Howard Fischer, "County Attorney Says Lawmakers Entitled to Ban Abortions at 20 Weeks," *Capitol News Services*, July 26, 2012, http://cvbugle.com/Main. asp?SectionID=1&SubSectionID=1&ArticleID=35423.

20. Robin Marty, "The Real Reason Anti-Choice Advocates Are Pushing Fetal Pain Laws," *Rewire.News*, May 30, 2011, https://rewire.news/article/2011/05/30/real-reason-antichoice-activists-pushing-fetal-pain-laws.

21. "Anti-Choice Arizona Legislators Push 'Medication Abortion Reversal' Amendment," *Rewire.News*, March 11, 2015, https://rewire.news/article/2015/03/11/anti-choice-arizona-legislators-push-medication-abortion-reversal-amendment.

22. Claire Landsbaum, "New Arizona Law Requires Doctors to Treat Fetuses 'Born Alive' During Abortions," *The Cut*, April 3, 2017, https://www.thecut.com/2017/04/arizona-governor-signs-restrictive-born-alive-abortion-law.html.

23. Anna North, "A Republican-Backed Bill to Protect "Abortion Survivors" Just Failed. It Still Matters." *Vox*, February 26, 2019, https://www.vox.com/policy-and-politics/2019/2/25/18239964/born-alive-abortion-survivors-protection-2019-sasse.

12: MISSISSIPPI

1. Emily Wagster Pettus and Laura Tillman, "New Law Targets Lone Abortion Clinic in Mississippi," *Daily Texan*, April 12, 2012, https://www.dailytexanonline.com/news/2012/04/13/new-law-targets-lone-abortion-clinic-in-miss.

2. Emily Wagster Pettus, "Mississippi 'Personhood' Amendment Vote Fails," Associated Press, November 8, 2011 http://www.huffingtonpost.com/2011/11/08/mississippi-personhood-amendment_n_1082546.html.

3. "Letter From Diane Derzis," www.wakeupmississippi.org, October 7, 2011.

4. Irin Carmon, "Personhood's Mississippi Moment of Truth," *Salon*, November 8, 2011, http://www.salon.com/2011/11/08/personhoods_mississippi_moment_of_truth.

5. Emily Wagster Pettus, "1 Abortion Reg Survives, 2 Die in Miss. Senate," Associated Press, April 3, 2012 http://www.necn.com/04/03/12/1-abortion-reg-survives-2-die-in-Miss-Se/landing_politics.html?&apID=dcd659638770487f811db1ad4f189b6d.

6. Kate Sheppard, "Abortion Foes Latest Backdoor Ban," *Mother Jones*, June 27, 2012, http://www.motherjones.com/politics/2011/06/abortion-foes-latest-backdoor-ban.

7. Emily Wagster Pettus, "Tate Reeves Blocking Nomination Because of Candidate's Ties to Abortion Clinic," Associated Press, April 24, 2012, http://www.10tv.com/content/stories/apexchange/2012/04/24/ms--mississippi-abortion.html.

8. Dr. Jen Gunter, "The medical nonsense and dangerous precedent of Mississippi's abortion bill HB 1390," Dr. Jen Gunter, June 29, 2012, http://drjengunter.wordpress.com/2012/06/29/the-medical-nonsense-and-terrible-precedent-of-mississippis-abortion-bill-hb-1390.

9. Pettus and Tillman, "New Law."

10. Laura Tillman, "Mississippi Senate Passes Abortion Regulation Bill," Associated Press, April 5, 2012, http://finance.yahoo.com/news/mississippi-senate-passes-abortion-regulation-125042579.html.

11. Laura Conaway, "Mississippi Lawmaker: Coat Hanger Abortions Might Come Back. 'But hey . . .'" *The Maddow Blog*, May 14, 2012, http://maddowblog.msnbc.com/_news/2012/05/14/11702049-mississippi-lawmaker-coat-hanger-abortions-might-come-back-but-hey?lite.

12. MJ Lee, "Bill Dooms Miss. Only Abortion Clinic," *Politico*, April 5, 2012, http://www.politico.com/news/stories/0412/74871.html.

13. Steven Ertelt, "Mississippi Could Become First Abortion-Free State," *Lifenews*, April 5, 2012, http://www.lifenews.com/2012/04/05/mississippi-could-become-first-abortion-free-state.

14. Esme Deprez and Elizabeth Waibel, "Mississippi May Be First U.S. State with No Abortion Clinic," *Bloomberg News*, June 22, 2012, http://www.businessweek.com/news/2012-06-22/mississippi-may-become-first-u-dot-s-dot-state-with-no-abortion-clinic.

15. Deprez and Waibel, "Mississippi May be First."

16. Emily Le Coz, "Update 1—Mississippi Sole Abortion Clinic Sues Over New Law," Reuters, June 27, 2012, http://in.reuters.com/article/2012/06/27/usa-abortion-mississippi-idINL2E8HRBZY20120627.

17. Center for Reproductive Rights, *Center for Reproductive Rights Takes Legal Action to Keep Last Abortion Clinic in Mississippi Open*, June 27, 2012.

18. "Center for Reproductive Rights Takes Legal Action."

19. CNN Wire Staff, "Mississippi Sole Abortion Clinic Can Stay Open, For Now," *CNN*, July 13, 2012, http://www.cnn.com/2012/07/13/justice/mississippi-abortion-clinic-ruling.

20. Interview, Michelle Mohaved, Center for Reproductive Rights, July 28, 2012.

21. Mississippi Department of Health, "Infant Mortality in Mississippi," http://msdh.ms.gov/msdhsite/_static/23,4569,266,291.html.

22. Interview, Dr. Willie Parker, July 24, 2012.

23. Women's Legislative Network of NCSL, National Conference of State Legislatures, http://www.ncsl.org/legislatures-elections/wln/women-in-state-legislatures-2011.aspx.

24. Interview, Pamela Merrit, July 22, 2012.

25. Emily Le Coz, "Abortion Clinic Gets Letter, Revocation Process Starts," *Jackson Clarion Ledger*, January 28, 2013, http://www.clarionledger.com/article/20130129/NEWS/301280034/Abortion-clinic-gets-letter-revocation-process-starts.

26. Robin Marty, "Despite Abortion Bans, TRAP Laws Are the Real Threat to Abortion Access in North Dakota," *Rewire.News*, March 26, 2013, https://rewire.news/article/2013/03/26/despite-abortion-bans-trap-law-is-the-real-threat-to-abortion-access-in-north-dakota.

27. Abigail Barnes, "Alabama Admitting Privileges Law Ruled Unconstitutional," National Women's Law Center, August 5, 2014, https://nwlc.org/blog/alabama-admitting-privileges-law-ruled-unconstitutional.

28. Anna North, "The Supreme Court Has Blocked a Louisiana Abortion Law—For Now," *Vox*, February 8, 2019, https://www.vox.com/2019/2/7/18215941/louisiana-abortion-law-supreme-court-admitting-privileges.

13: "THE BURDEN IS UNDUE"

1. Manny Fernandez, "Filibuster in Texas Senate Tries to Halt Abortion Bill," *New York Times*, June 25, 2013, https://www.nytimes.com/2013/06/26/us/politics/senate-democrats-in-texas-try-blocking-abortion-bill-with-filibuster.html.

2. Margaret Hartmann, "Dramatic Filibuster Beats Texas Anti-Abortion Bill (Eventually)," *New York*, June 26, 2013, http://nymag.com/intelligencer/2013/06/filibuster-beats-texas-abortion-bill.html?gtm=bottom.

3. Manny Fernandez, "Abortion Restrictions Become Law in Texas, but Opponents Will Press Fight," *New York Times*, July 18, 2013, https://www.nytimes.com/2013/07/19/us/perry-signs-texas-abortion-restrictions-into-law.html.

4. Sarah Mervosh, "Dallas Doctors Settle with Hospital, Can Continue Doing Abortions," *Dallas Morning News*, June 9, 2014 https://www.dallasnews.com/news/news/2014/06/09/dallas-doctors-settle-with-hospital-can-continue-doing-abortions.

5. Candice Russell, "Women Already Have to Travel Across the Country to Get Abortions. I Was One of Them," *Glamour*, November 28, 2016, https://www.glamour.com/story/i-went-across-the-country-for-my-abortion.

6. Alexa Ura, "Judge Strikes Down Texas Abortion Regulation," *Texas Tribune*, August 29, 2014, https://www.texastribune.org/2014/08/29/federal-judge-strikes-down-texas-abortion-regulati.

7. Lauren Gambino, "Appeals Court Allows Texas to Enforce Controversial Anti-Abortion Law," *The Guardian*, October 2, 2014, https://www.theguardian.com/world/2014/oct/02/appeals-court-texas-abortion-law.

8. Robin Marty, "This Lawyer Fought to Keep the Texas Abortion Clinics Open," *Cosmopolitan*, October 3, 2014, https://www.cosmopolitan.com/politics/news/a31766/brigitte-amiri-aclu-texas-abortion-clinics.

9. Adam Liptak, "Supreme Court Allows Texas Abortion Clinics to Stay Open," *New York Times*, October 14, 2014, https://www.nytimes.com/2014/10/15/us/supreme-court-allows-texas-abortion-clinics-to-stay-open.html.

10. Manny Fernandez and Erik Eckholm, "Court Upholds Texas Limits on Abortions," *New York Times*, June 9, 2015, https://www.nytimes.com/2015/06/10/us/court-upholds-texas-law-criticized-as-blocking-access-to-abortions.html.

11. Oral arguments, Whole Woman's Health et al v. Hellerstedt, March 2, 2016, https://www.reproductiverights.org/sites/crr.civicactions.net/files/documents/WholeWomansHealthvHellerstedt-Oral-Argument-Transcript-15-274_l53m.pdf.

12. Ibid.

13. Whole Woman's Health et al. V. Hellerstedt, Commissioner, Texas Department of State Health Services, et al. Certiorari to the united states court of appeals for the fifth circuit No. 15–274. Argued March 2, 2016—Decided June 27, 2016. https://www.supremecourt.gov/opinions/15pdf/15-274_new_e18f.pdf.

14. Molly Redden, "Planned Parenthood: Eight States Now Striving to Repeal Abortion Restrictions," *The Guardian*, June 30, 2016, https://www.theguardian.com/us-news/2016/jun/30/planned-parenthood-state-repeal-abortion-restrictions.

14: INTO THE TRUMP YEARS

1. Susan B. Anthony List, "Trump Outlines Pro-Life Commitments, Taps SBA List's Dannenfelser to Chair Pro-Life Coalition," September 16, 2016, https://www.sba-list.org/newsroom/press-releases/trump-outlines-pro-life-commitments-taps-sba-lists-dannenfelser-chair-pro-life-coalition.

2. Jessica Martínez and Gregory A. Smith, "How the Faithful Voted: A Preliminary 2016 Analysis," Pew Research Center, November 9, 2016. https://www.pewresearch.org/fact-tank/2016/11/09/how-the-faithful-voted-a-preliminary-2016-analysis.

3. Interview with Mary Alice Carter, April 10, 2019.

4. "Strategic Plan," U.S. Department of Health and Human Services, last reviewed on February 28, 2018, https://www.hhs.gov/about/strategic-plan/introduction/index.html#organizational.

5. Carter Sherman, "Exclusive: Trump Officials Discussed "Reversing" Abortion for Undocumented Teen," *VICE News*, January 31, 2018 https://news.vice.com/en_us/article/yw5a5g/exclusive-trump-officials-discussed-reversing-abortion-for-undocumented-teen.

6. Stacy Sullivan, "Jane Doe Wants an Abortion But the Government Is Hellbent on Stopping Her," ACLU, October 19, 2017, https://www.aclu.org/blog/immigrants-rights/immigrants-rights-and-detention/jane-doe-wants-abortion-government-hell-bent.

7. Robert Barnes and Ann E. Marimow, "Supreme Court Throws Out Lower-Court Decision that Allowed Immigrant Teen to Obtain Abortion," *Washington Post*, June 4, 2018, https://www.washingtonpost.com/politics/courts_law/supreme-court-throws-out-lower-court-decision-that-allowed-immigrant-teenager-to-obtain-abortion/2018/06/04/50a59ba4-67f5-11e8-bea7-c8eb28bc52b1_story.html?utm_term=.96b60faf0126.

8. Ema O'Connor. "A Judge Just Ruled That The Trump Administration Cannot Block Undocumented Pregnant Teens From Getting Abortions," *Buzzfeed*, March 30, 2018, https://www.buzzfeednews.com/article/emaoconnor/trump-administration-cannot-block-undocumented-teens.

9. "Compliance With Statutory Program Intergrity Requirements," 84 *Federal Register* 42, March 4, 2019, p. 7714, https://www.govinfo.gov/content/pkg/FR-2019-03-04/pdf/2019-03461.pdf.

10. "Congress Didn't Defund Planned Parenthood. But Trump Can," *Washington Update*, Family Research Council, March 29, 2018, https://www.frc.org/washingtonupdate/20180329/congress-defund.

11. Obria Group, "HHS Awards Obria Group $5.1 Million in Title X Family Planning Grants" March 30, 2019, https://obriagroup.org/hhs-awards-title-x.

12. "Birth Control," Obria Medical Clinics, https://www.obria.org/birth-control.

13. Matt Hadro, "Trump's Executive Order Praised as Key 'First Step' Protecting Religious Freedom," *National Catholic Register*, May 4, 2017, http://www.ncregister.com/daily-news/trumps-executive-order-praised-as-key-first-step-protecting-religious-freed.

14. "President Donald J. Trump stands up for religious freedom in the United

States," May 3, 2018, https://www.whitehouse.gov/briefings-statements/president-donald-j-trump-stands-religious-freedom-united-states.

15. "Attorney General Sessions Delivers Remarks at the Department of Justice's Religious Liberty Summit, Washington, DC," Monday, July 30, 2018 https://www.justice.gov/opa/speech/attorney-general-sessions-delivers-remarks-department-justice-s-religious-liberty-summit.

16. Jessica Ravitz, "Online Abortion Pill Provider Ordered to Cease Delivery by FDA," *CNN*, March 17, 2019, https://www.cnn.com/2019/03/15/health/fda-aid-access-abortion-pill-warning/index.html.

17. "Violence Statistics and History," National Abortion Federation, https://prochoice.org/education-and-advocacy/violence/violence-statistics-and-history/ accessed April 4, 2019.

18. FACE, Department of Justice, https://www.justice.gov/crt/special-litigation-section-cases-and-matters0#face accessed April 4, 2019.

19. Carole Novielli, "10 Pro-Life Activists Charged Under the Federal F.A.C.E. Act," *Live Action*, July 19, 2017, https://www.liveaction.org/news/pro-life-activists-charged-face-act.

20. Nina Liss-Schultz, "The Militant Wing of the Anti-Abortion Movement Is Back—And It's Never Been Closer to Victory," *Mother Jones*, September/October 2018, https://www.motherjones.com/crime-justice/2018/09/abortion-clinic-blockade-red-rose-rescue.

15: HOW THE TRIGHT WON THE JUDICIARY

1. Philip Bump, "A Quarter of Republicans Voted for Trump to get Supreme Court Picks—and It Paid Off," *Washington Post*, June 26, 2018, https://www.washingtonpost.com/news/politics/wp/2018/06/26/a-quarter-of-republicans-voted-for-trump-to-get-supreme-court-picks-and-it-paid-off/?utm_term=.436f83286f4b.

2. Burwell v. Hobby Lobby Stores, June 30, 2014, https://www.oyez.org/cases/2013/13-354.

3. Andrew Cohen, "The Most Conservative Supreme Court in History Will Move Further Right," *Rolling Stone*, June 27, 2018, https://www.rollingstone.com/politics/politics-news/the-most-conservative-supreme-court-in-a-century-will-move-further-right-666869.

4. Garza v. Hargan, Millett dissent, https://www.cadc.uscourts.gov/internet/opinions.nsf/C81A5EDEADAE82F2852581C30068AF6E/$file/17-5236-1701167.pdf.

5. Sophie Tatum, "Brett Kavanaugh's Nomination: A Timeline," *CNN Poltics*, accessed April 7, 2019, https://www.cnn.com/interactive/2018/10/politics/timeline-kavanaugh.

6. "Brett Kavanaugh's Attack on Democrats Could Pose Risk to Supreme Court," *CBS News*, September 29, 2018, https://www.cbsnews.com/news/brett-kavanaugh-attack-on-democrats-poses-risk-to-supreme-court.

7. National Right to Life, *Groundbreaking Dismemberment Abortion Ban in Kansas Leads Off Right to Life Movement 2015 Lesgislative Agenda*, January 14, 2015, https://webcache.googleusercontent.com/search?q=cache:dVZKku1-1MsJ:https://www.nrlc.org/communications/releases/2015/release011415/+&cd=1&hl=en&ct=clnk&gl=us&client=firefox-b-1-d.

8. Kansas SB 95, 2015 Session http://kslegislature.org/li_2016/b2015_16/measures/documents/sb95_00_0000.pdf.

9. Testimony of Anthony Levatino, MD, JD, before the Kansas Senate Health & Human Services Committee, February 2, 2015, http://kslegislature.org/li_2016/b2015_16/committees/ctte_s_phw_1/documents/testimony/20150202_08.pdf.

10. Robin Marty, "Kansas Legislator Dick Jones Uses Every Abortion Trope in Just One Hearing," Care2, March 10, 2015, https://www.care2.com/causes/kansas-legislator-dick-jones-uses-every-abortion-trope-in-just-one-hearing.html.

11. Ryan Newton, "Governor to Re-enact Signing of Anti-Abortion Measure," KSNW.com, April 27, 2015, https://www.ksn.com/news/local/governor-to-re-enact-signing-of-anti-abortion-measure/1023458588.

12. "Bans on Specific Abortion Methods Used After the First Trimester," Guttmacher Institute, https://www.guttmacher.org/state-policy/explore/bans-specific-abortion-methods-used-after-first-trimester.

13. Marshall v. West Alabama Women's Center amicus brief, https://www.supremecourt.gov/DocketPDF/18/18-837/86943/20190204155739057_18-837%20Amicus%20Brief%20Louisiana--PDFA.pdf.

14. Natasha Bach, "Most Americans Want Roe v. Wade to Stay, According to New Poll," Fortune, September 12, 2018, http://fortune.com/2018/09/12/roe-v-wade-poll-abortion.

16: WHERE IT ALL ENDS

1. U.S. Senate, Pain-Capable Unborn Child Protection Act, S.160, 116th Congress, Introduced January 16, 2019, https://www.congress.gov/bill/116th-congress/senate-bill/160/text.

2. "Fact Sheet: The Science of Fetal Pain," Charlotte Lozier Institute, https://lozierinstitute.org/fact-sheet-science-of-fetal-pain.

3. Alex Swoyer, "Senate Republicans Note Fetal Pain Threshold in 20 Week in Effort to Ban Abortion After 20 Weeks," Washington Times, April 9, 2019, https://www.washingtontimes.com/news/2019/apr/9/20-week-abortion-ban-bill-notes-fetal-pain-thresho.

4. Sarah G. Miller, "Do Fetuses Feel Pain? What the Science Says," Live Science, May 17, 2016, https://www.livescience.com/54774-fetal-pain-anesthesia.html.

5. 4.9.19 Senate Judiciary Hearing on Pain Capable bill, Dr. Donna Harrison Testimony, https://www.youtube.com/watch?v=XGqPq-lRIRE.